# AUTISTIC ADULTS

# AUTISTIC ADULTS

## Exploring the Forgotten End of the Spectrum

DANIEL SMEENK

Ronsdale Press

AUTISTIC ADULTS



RONSDALE PRESS
125A – 1030 Denman Street, Vancouver, B.C. Canada V6G 2M6
www.ronsdalepress.com

Book Design: Derek von Essen
Cover Design: David Lester

Ronsdale Press wishes to thank the following for their support of its publishing program: the Canada Council for the Arts, the Government of Canada, the British Columbia Arts Council, and the Province of British Columbia through the British Columbia Book Publishing Tax Credit program.

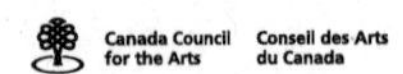

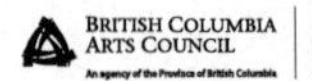

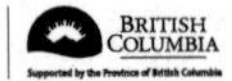

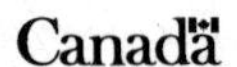


LIBRARY AND ARCHIVES CANADA CATALOGUING IN PUBLICATION

Title: Autistic adults : exploring the forgotten end of the spectrum / Daniel Smeenk.
Names: Smeenk, Daniel, author.
Description: Includes index.
Identifiers: Canadiana (print) 2023047716X | Canadiana (ebook) 20230477178 | ISBN 9781553806950 (softcover) | ISBN 9781553806974 (PDF) | ISBN 9781553806967 (EPUB)
Subjects: LCSH: Autistic people. | LCSH: Autism.
Classification: LCC RC553.A88 S64 2023 | DDC 616.85/882—dc23

At Ronsdale Press we are committed to protecting the environment. To this end we are working with Canopy and printers to phase out our use of paper produced from ancient forests. This book is one step towards that goal.

PRINTED IN CANADA

Dedicated to my uncle,
Douglas Gunter

## CONTENTS

## ACKNOWLEDGEMENTS

The heart of this book are the people who agreed to be interviewed, especially the twenty-three autistic adults and four parents of autistic adults who shared their experiences between January and August 2021. They made this book not just possible but meaningful.

The demographics for the autistic interviewees break down like this: eleven people were over forty and twelve people were under forty; there were ten men, twelve women, and one person who identified as non-binary; and there were eight Canadians, eight Americans, three people from the U.K. (two from England and one in Northern Ireland), and one person each from India, New Zealand, Israel, and Belgium.

In the interest of full disclosure, Todd Simkover, Noam Grossman, and Thomas Yackimec were friends before I started on this book. Jacob Dean is a second cousin. Everyone else came forward through requests made to non-profit organizations, particularly Autism Canada, Action for Autism, which is based in India, and the Asperger/Autism Network (AANE).

Three of the autistic people I interviewed requested anonymity. It has been given to them.

I also found people willing to be interviewed on the Facebook groups Autistic Not Weird and Autistic Researchers Researching Autism. I am very thankful to these groups and their members who agreed to be interviewed.

Among the people I interviewed, three are self-diagnosed. To not single them out, I haven't named them in this book. I mention this because self-diagnosis is a controversial topic. People in the autistic self-advocacy community tend to accept self-diagnosis, while those outside of it tend to be more skeptical.

To receive services, I think people need an official diagnosis from a qualified professional, and I believe there is no substitute for one. I highly recommend anyone who may be autistic to seek a diagnosis. As a matter of personal identity, which was what interested me for this book, I accept self-diagnosis because there is typically no advantage to it, especially given the stigma that still exists with autism. It's also often the first step on an important journey.

An assessment can involve a long waiting list and a lot of money, which is why people are sometimes slow to get one. They can quite reasonably believe they are autistic, however, especially if they have realized this as an adult. I believe everyone I interviewed for the book is autistic. You can decide whether you want to believc that everyone, including self-diagnosed people, are autistic.

There were also ten other on-the-record interviews represent a wide swath of the autism community, from professionals to academics to non-profit workers. They all represented different points of view, which were equally valuable for my own understanding of the world of autism.

I also had many off-the-record conversations with professionals and researchers who really helped me understand these issues better. Some of these conversations were made after reaching out through email, and some came from connections made at conferences.

I am thankful to the professionals at the National Autism Conference at Penn State who helped me understand behaviourism better. I am also thankful to the autistic people at the Aucademy Autistic Mental Health and Well-Being conference and the Participatory Autism Research Collective's Critical Autism Studies conference for better-understanding autism as seen by other autistic people.

I am also hugely thankful to Martin Wightman and Judith Brand for editing this book, as well as Dr. Jason Travers at Temple University for providing a very needed expert opinion. I would also like to thank Bruce Petherick for giving me an interview, and for providing a well-informed autistic perspective that gave me insight into the entire book.

Of course, I would also like to thank Ronsdale Press for publishing this book. I did not write this book with the expectation that a publisher would agree to publish it. You have helped spread this message more than I could have ever reasonably hoped to.

I'm also grateful for the numerous friends and family who read drafts and gave me feedback. Apart from their wise and trusted advice, they also reflect the people I am writing this book for in many ways, so their advice was particularly appreciated.

## DISCLAIMER ON QUOTES AND LANGUAGE

THE QUOTES FROM THE AUTISTIC ADULTS and parents of autistic adults were approved before publication by those who said them.

This is not a typical practice of journalistic writing. I do not usually condone this practice, as you can sometimes end up being a mouthpiece for the source and lose your independence and objectivity. I felt in this case, however, that the benefits outweighed the drawbacks.

These are not people who have something to gain through giving interviews. They are sharing deeply personal stories. The risk of making an error and publicly misrepresenting them outweighed the perceived loss of independence on my part. I also do not believe in this case that the message or the material would be fundamentally changed by their approval or disapproval. Nevertheless, this fact should be understood by the audience before reading this book.

I did not offer the same privilege to people who were interviewed for their expertise. I am deeply grateful for their participation, and I hope and believe that I will represent them and their work accurately. But the stakes are different. They are not pouring out sensitive details of their lives.

I also want to make some notes on language. This is one of the most contentious issues in the world of autism. The difference between language in and out of the autistic community is stark and often not used without meaningful consequences. Using some language will offend the autistic community; using other language can be confusing and jargony for people outside the community.

In general, I will use the terms that are preferred by the autistic self-advocacy community. I will say "autistic people" rather than "person with autism." I will say someone "is autistic" rather than "has autism." I will refer to "autism spectrum condition" or "on the autism spectrum," and not "autism spectrum disorder" except in explicit references to the *Diagnostic and Statistical Manual* (DSM) or in quotes.

I will refer to support needs rather than functioning labels ("low support needs" rather than "high functioning") if I must refer to an autistic person's support needs at all. I will refer to "traits" and not "symptoms." I will say "non-speaking" rather than "non-verbal."

Similarly, I will be more likely to use words like "more obvious" rather than "severe" to describe an autistic person's outward presentation. This one might be a little controversial, but I feel that distinguishing between autistic people who present differently is a must, and this was the clearest and least offensive term I could come up with.

While there may be similar challenges at some level, my life and the life of an autistic person who does not speak are quite different in meaningful ways.

I also usually say that an autistic person "can" have a particular trait, rather than autistic people "do" have a trait. Autistic people are significantly different from each other. It rarely makes sense to say that autistic people are all one way or another. This book will look at trends, not absolutes. When the topic is autism, absolute statements are often impossible to make.

Most importantly, I will use "neurotypical" rather than "normal." Neurotypical simply refers to people who are non-autistic, but in neurodiversity circles, it can also mean people who do not have other developmental or learning conditions, such as attention deficit hyperactivity disorder (ADHD) or dyslexia. For those unfamiliar with neurodiversity circles, neurotypical is a neutral descriptive term. It's not a bad thing to be neurotypical.

Referring to neurotypicals as "normal," which has been standard for a lot of the history of autism, implies autistic people are abnormal. This makes many people feel stigmatized. I have no desire to offend or provoke discomfort.

I have stronger personal feelings about some of these terms than others, but the autistic community is understandably sensitive about this in a way that is not equivalent among researchers, professionals, or even family members. I also do not believe using these terms takes away from any truth I wish to present in this book.

There are some language practices of the self-advocacy community I will not use. Some members of the community capitalize Autism and Autistic, as a way of signifying they are talking about an identity rather than an adjective for a person. I feel that this is too jarring and esoteric for a broader audience and is much more entrenched within the autistic community than outside. I will use the lower case "autism" or "autistic."

I have also italicized sections of the book that contain practical advice for neurotypical people. I am grateful to my editor and others who read the book in advance for emphasizing a need to stress practical advice in this book. This gives a purpose to the theoretical discussion essential to setting up the foundation for this advice.

I hope the reader will examine the context as well, as it is essential to understanding why the practical advice matters. I hope this format makes the take-aways clear.

# INTRODUCTION

MY MOM HAS TOLD ME THIS STORY since I was young.

When I was two years old, myself, my parents, and my then-in-utero sister were in Indonesia because of my father's work at an American engineering firm.

My father, who is a Dutch-descended Canadian, played soccer on a team of Dutch internationals in a local recreational soccer league. This brought me to soccer games played against other teams of other international residents.

At the time, and sometimes still today, I was often noticing less of the game and more of the small details of interest to me. On this day, I was particularly interested in the numbers on the players' backs. By this age, I had already started to read in English and could sound out words in both English and Bahasa Indonesian.[1]

I looked at one of the players' backs, where I saw their jersey number was nineteen, and I said out loud, "Nineteen," and then, "sembilan belas," which is the same number in Indonesian. Overhearing this, a woman came over to my mom and asked her how old I was. When my mom replied, the woman remarked how unusual it was for someone my age to know a number that high in two different languages.

This was an aha moment for my mom. I was different. Noticing these sorts of small details is a classic sign of a way of thinking called autism.

Within a year of this conversation at the soccer game, I got a diagnosis of pervasive developmental disorder — not otherwise specified (PDD-NOS), a now-defunct diagnosis that was incorporated into a broad autism spectrum disorder in 2013. This PDD-NOS diagnosis was later changed to Asperger's syndrome when I was eleven, another autism-related diagnosis absorbed under the broad autism umbrella.

This diagnosis, and the traits it describes, has affected my life, my identity, and my outlook on the world.

These diagnoses were reflective not just of odd skills like being able to count high but also of more irritating traits to others. I was an abnormally picky eater, who at the age of three would only eat white-coloured foods like potatoes and meats. Even to this day, certain foods, like most fruits and especially bananas, can be deeply unsettling to even smell, never mind eat.

Once I started school, my attention and hyperactivity became an issue and a distraction, and I was even put on Ritalin (which didn't work). I was a nice kid whom teachers liked, but I had difficulty making friends my own age. On one day, I could recite dozens of statistics from memory to the astonishment of my classmates and adults; another day, I was sitting alone at recess or being teased for jumping up and down and flapping my arms repeatedly, one of my "stims" displayed during my excited periods.

Due to the attentiveness and proactiveness of my parents, however, there was not a time in my life that I did not know that I was autistic and, therefore, why all this was happening. This part of my identity predates almost everything else about me, from my strong interests in music, history, and politics to a consciousness of my moodiness and chatty nature, especially when comfortable and on a topic of interest.

Autism likely influenced all of this. It is the oldest and most constant part of my identity.

There is a lot of literature about people like my three- or even ten-year-old self, but these young, different children eventually grow up, like anyone else — and they're still autistic. This part of autism — the adult part — has seldom been written about, especially in a comprehensive and systematic way for a general audience.

That's where this book comes in.

In part 1, I will talk about the history and basic traits of autistic adults. I will look at autism's two core diagnostic criteria from the perspective of clinicians, parents of autistic adults, and autistic adults themselves. You will, I hope, start to get to know autistic adults and understand their lives after finishing this section.

In part 2, I look at four personal and societal challenges that autistic adults face. These are issues with lack of data, lack of resources and employment, lack of understanding from society, and lack of understanding of themselves, especially given the messages autistic people often get from others within neurotypical society.

This book may be of interest to autistic people, researchers, and professionals. Much of the information in this book will be less likely to be new for these groups, but its comprehensiveness means even they may learn something.

Mainly, this book is written for neurotypicals — those who are not autistic. This is the most important group in autistic adults' day-to-day lives. They are who autistic people are most likely to interact with in their families, at the grocery store, or in their jobs. This is the group that needs to hear their stories the most, because they often have the most impact on an autistic person's well-being.

The person I imagine may get something out of this book is the person who knows an autistic adult in their life. Maybe they work with autistic colleagues or they manage autistic people, and they hope to get them more involved in social activities or help them be less anxious at work. Maybe they are interested in policy and hope to learn something about broad issues surrounding autistic adults because of the implications on their work.

A person coming in with these kinds of motivations will get something out of this book.

I hope this book is accessible to everyone, while also reflecting the current state of the scholarly literature. Because I know a lot of different kinds of people may read this book, it cannot be assumed they know about the autism community. There are some important things to know about it.

Autism is a fractious field with many controversies. There are many different people with different interests. They do not just have different opinions about particulars, but different worldviews about what autism is and means.

One of the autistic people I interviewed told me that there was a major divergence between the "autism community" and the "autistic community." This is a commonly understood dynamic within the autism world that is essential to understanding the rest of this book.

By "autism community," what's generally included in this group are neurotypical parents of autistic people and certain academics and researchers, especially those who are not autistic themselves and who follow a more classic understanding of autism. Long-established organizations like the Autism Society of America, the many parents who volunteer with groups like Autism Speaks, and some mainstream child psychologists are generally seen as subscribing to this kind of view, even if they wouldn't describe themselves this way.

This group broadly supports behaviourist schools of thought and follows the "medical model of disability," which sees autism as something as much to manage and treat than nurture and embrace.

A practitioner of a behaviourist-based therapy emphasized to me that their approach is not medical, in that they do not see behaviour as part of an illness and also look at their environment. While this is important to keep in mind, members of the autism community are nevertheless often seen as more likely to support both behaviourism and the medical model rather than one or the other.

There can be some nurturing and kindness involved in this approach. Most people in the autism community do not dislike autistic people and hope to retain qualities in them that they believe will not hurt them.

Nevertheless, the belief in helping autistic people to better fit into society is their key focus. They do this by teaching them the skills necessary to avoid stigmatization, such as how to look people in the eye or how to have reciprocal conversation. To the autistic community, they can see at least some autistic traits as something that will hold autistic people back from fulfilling their potential, as well as make them more dependent on others. They believe this is the best way to make autistic people's lives easier.

The criticism of this approach usually comes from the "autistic community." These are usually autistic adolescents and adults who believe in the idea of neurodiversity, a movement that believes autism is one form of how brains are wired — as valid as a neurotypical brain.

The autistic community also tends to embrace some form or another of what is called the "social model of disability," which refers to the way that society disables people by setting up institutions that don't fit their needs. A paraplegic is more disabled if they do not have ramps and elevators, for example, and autistic people can be more disadvantaged when there is too much sensory overload somewhere they should be able to access, or social communication demands are too overly complex.

Someone in the autism community might deal with this situation by helping the autistic person find ways to cope, such as bringing noise-cancelling headphones to those sensitive to loud noise. A person in the autistic community is more likely to question why the world is so loud to begin with and more likely to focus on making malls and supermarkets quieter, which they argue would benefit everyone.

Throughout this book, I will also sometimes refer to this community as the "self-advocacy community." This is a way to distinguish between autistic people active in neurodiversity communities and autistic people who are not involved in these communities, whatever their beliefs might be.

Just as not all autistic people think the same, there are also some parents, researchers, and professionals who subscribe to something more like the social model of disability and neurodiversity.

The perspective of both groups is essential to understanding the world of autism. Many parents and clinicians have a perspective of looking after a more obviously autistic person, someone who requires a high amount of attention and care to get through life.

In contrast, the self-advocacy community often brings the perspective of less obviously presenting adults. The autistic community, therefore, tends to look at issues through this experience.

Both the autistic and autism communities' perspectives make sense given their fundamental assumptions and starting points.

I interviewed people who broadly represent both communities in this book. I read the writings of both and talked to some people who do not cleanly fit either description. I believe the moderate wings of both communities have good intentions and have strengths and weaknesses in their approaches. In many ways, they are also not mutually exclusive. Throughout this book, it will be clear that there are areas that both communities commonly see as meaningful.

However, both communities tend to dislike each other, which can sometimes lead to expectations that a book like this will represent one side or the other. As an autistic person, I see the autistic community perspective more readily, but if anyone from either community is looking for me to be their voice, they are reading the wrong book.

I come to very few absolute conclusions or recommendations in this book, particularly because of the high stakes and the controversial nature of the subject. This is not an advocacy book at its heart. With my background as a non-expert, I feel I would do more harm than good trying to provide too much strong advocacy on policy and autism research especially.

I wrote this as a way of presenting the issues to someone who may have never really engaged with them, while not strongly advocating for one side or another.

The recommendations that I do come to in this book are largely to find points of agreement between the autism and autistic communities, as I do believe this will be necessary in the long run for the well-being of everyone in both communities.

*I certainly do not recommend any sort of medical treatment in this book.*

What I *do* try to do is to explore these topics, both at a factual and an emotional level. I try to make them understandable to a layperson. If people who subscribe to various perspectives believe I have done them justice, then I feel I have done my job.

A reader may also notice a largely North American bias to this book. This is mainly related to the fact that I'm Canadian, live in Canada, and have direct experience with how autism is treated in North America. I simply understand it the best.

This bias, for instance, will mean there is much more attention to the *Diagnostic and Statistical Manual* rather than the *International Classification of Diseases*, which is more often used in Europe. Many global studies are cited, but most of the information centres on North American research and institutions. The people I interviewed were also mostly but not solely from North America.

While there are cultural and economic differences that affect autistic people, the autistic experience has similarities everywhere, so I hope people from around the world reading this can find something that is useful to them.

As a note to autistic people, nothing in this book should be taken as meaning something specific to them. A major criticism of current autism research from the self-advocacy community is that it tends to approach autism as a pathology first, without seeing life from an autistic person's point of view. This is often seen as disrespectful of an autistic person and may make them feel personally attacked, with a common response being something like "I'm autistic and I'm not like that."

I understand this criticism on a deeply personal level. I do write about some of the broad downsides of autism in this book because they exist and should be talked about, and some people may take this personally. If they read that something applies to a lot of people but know it does not apply to them, they should trust their own intuition before my words.

If this book helps an autistic person feel better and understand themselves, as I suspect some parts might, that is a welcome by-product. When talking about the tendencies of any group, there will always be exceptions, especially with autistic people.

The story of autistic adults is one that has been seldom told. Autistic adults have created a lively community, which despite serious divisions is a wonderful place overall, and their stories and traits deserve to be understood by the whole society. Growing up as an autistic person brings with it an experience of life as full as anyone else's — in some ways maybe even just a little bit more.

I hope the reader will get a glimpse of that story in this book.

# PART 1

# CHAPTER 1:
# A HISTORY AND OVERVIEW OF AUTISM

TO UNDERSTAND AUTISTIC ADULTS, it's important to understand autism itself. Autism is best viewed as both a disability community and a culture. Although they should both be equally kept in mind, let's start with the disability aspect as it provides the basics.

Autism is a genetically based developmental condition that is also influenced by environmental factors. Autism is always present from birth, but a diagnosis can usually be reliably made when the person is around eighteen months old. A diagnosis at two years old is considered "very reliable."[1]

What does a "developmental condition" mean? This means autism affects how a person's brain develops throughout the course of their life. The simplest way to explain this is by comparing a neurotypical person's life to an autistic person's.

A neurotypical person is more likely to make verbal sounds by twelve to eighteen months old; read and write at age five; make friends in childhood; have a romantic relationship in their teens and get married and have kids in adulthood.[2] Of course, not everyone follows this path exactly. However, those who don't do it for reasons other than having a developmental condition. They can do this out of choice, like being in the clergy and taking a vow of celibacy, or they could also do this because of mental or physical trauma, which can affect people's perceptions and abilities.

For autistic people, if they make these milestones at all, they are more likely to be unconventional in how and when they do meet them. This is because of challenges they have in doing so that are directly related to their neurological development.

Autism is diagnosed by a psychologist through studied observations of behaviour and often other assessments, which can include interviewing family or close friends or hearing tests to rule out deafness as a cause of speech difficulties.[3]

The psychologist is guided by criteria in the 5th edition of the *Diagnostic and Statistical Manual*, often shortened to DSM, to make a diagnosis. Two core DSM criteria form "autism spectrum disorder," as the official diagnosis is called: current or past issues with "social communication" and "restricted and repetitive behaviours."

"Social communication" has three subcategories, as quoted in the DSM: difficulty holding a conversation, issues with non-verbal communication, and problems forming and maintaining friendships. "Restricted and repetitive behaviours" has four: unusual repeated self-soothing activities, such as rocking back and forth; strict routines; intensely focused topics of interest; and issues with the sensory environment, which include sounds being too loud, sights being too bright, or tastes being too intense.

A person must have both core criteria to be diagnosed as autistic. They also must have all three social communication subcategories and at least two of the four restricted and repetitive behaviours.[4] After being diagnosed, the person is often assigned at Level 1, 2, or 3. These levels refer to how much external support they will likely need to manage day-to-day life, with 1 being the least and 3 being the most.

In general, Level 1 requires "support," meaning a person may need some assistance with specific skills, like holding a conversation or keeping on task at school or work. They may need some therapy or training to help them with these skills. Sometimes that isn't always necessary as people at Level 1 might not even notice their own autism and it can go unnoticed by others.

It is not unusual for people at Level 1 to attain normal milestones. People who were diagnosed with a prior label called Asperger's syndrome, which later merged into autism, often fall into this category. The criteria for diagnosing Asperger's syndrome were that they talked within the expected age range, were potty trained within the normal range, and had normal or above-normal intelligence. It's often the social skills and ways of coping with the world that are different.[5]

Level 2 requires "substantial support," where autism becomes more obvious to laypeople and can mean a more constant relationship with caretakers, support workers, and services. People at this level may have issues with engaging in the outside world, such as a limited speaking vocabulary, intellectual disability, or highly structured routines that can cause meltdowns if even slightly altered.

Level 3 requires "very substantial support," which often means being completely non-speaking, needing round-the-clock care, and even more clear and obvious difficulties in the two core areas.[6]

At both Levels 2 and 3, there is a more complicated pattern of development. Sometimes kids at these levels are late at learning skills if they learn them at all. Sometimes they acquire skills early in life and then lose them. Usually, it all happens within the toddler stage, about eighteen months to two years.[7]

These categories are not absolutes. A person can have a single profound difficulty that really impacts their overall development but exhibit multiple other areas of real strength. Whatever classification a person is given is best decided by a psychologist doing an evaluation, and an assessment of an autistic person later in life might change that classification, reflecting how that person develops.

The entirety of this look at autism is also purely clinical, which has a lot of use, but it also does not tell the whole story.

## An Incomplete Picture

Anyone who has been around autism even a little knows that quoting the DSM barely begins to capture what it truly is.

Special education teacher and prominent autistic self-advocate Stephen Shore is famous for saying, "If you've met one person with autism, you've met one person with autism."[8] If it is known that a person is autistic, this means they likely deal with some challenges that neurotypical people do not, but little more can be assumed than that.

The risk in ordinary life is that the autism diagnosis can override everything else about that person. The diagnosis does not say whether a person is friendly, grumpy, intelligent, or funny. An autistic person can be all these things depending on the moment, and their overall personality significantly changes the quality of their life.

It is also not inherently prescriptive of their future. An autism diagnosis likely means that certain parts of life are a challenge, sometimes a really significant one, but it does not say how they live up to their potential as workers, friends, or family. *In short, being autistic is not the end of the world.*

This is where a double standard can come in since a neurotypical person is not generally as starkly labelled on their own limitations, such as quickness to anger, greed, or other faults. These can be deep issues that affect their life, even if they are not diagnosable as autistic. In this respect and others, autistic people are not judged by the same standards as neurotypicals.

Most neurotypicals also have these assumptions about what the label of autism means, which can be completely wrong. To take merely one example, despite the old stereotype of autistic people being introverted loners, social communication differences are not always about autistic people withdrawing from others. While some autistic people are more withdrawn, or at least only willing to talk to certain people (selective mutism), social communication issues also include what clinicians call an "active but odd" personality type.[9] These people can be gregarious and outgoing, often with good intentions, but may not understand how to engage in a way that is familiar and reassuring to others. This lack of understanding of other people can lead them to be misunderstood, themselves.

The DSM criteria also does not account for skills that come to autistic people at all levels. Dr. Temple Grandin, an autistic pioneer whose early childhood was in the 1950s, would likely be considered obviously autistic by today's standards. She did not speak until age four, and her mother was even given a recommendation that she be institutionalized. With help, however, particularly from her mother and an influential science teacher, she learned enough skills to interact with most people, and to speak and write well, while not being any less autistic. She became an accomplished academic researcher in animal science and is now world-famous for her cattle chute designs.

Grandin attributes this skill to being able to think like the cattle, which is not a scientifically demonstrated trait among autistic people but may be a noteworthy insight.[10] Despite her considerable career accomplishments, she has never had a romantic partner due to the social demands of such a relationship.[11] This would make many neurotypical people miserable, and some would consider those who are not in these relationships as being somehow broken. But Grandin is a highly accomplished person whose life appears happy despite this. Autistic lives like Grandin's can sometimes reveal the troubles with conventional measures of success. For some people, unconventional paths may be their best course through life.

This is also where the problem with labels such as "high" and "low" functioning, which are commonly used among both academics and laypeople but are often loathed in the autistic community. Attaching a label like "low functioning" brings low expectations onto people who can be capable of much more than what someone superficially sees. With proper support, an autistic person may not have a neurotypical's life, nor should they necessarily hope for one, but they can learn skills to help find their own way to a happy life.

The opposite problems can come to a person with Level 1 autism. Some people still think that autism is a condition that is always obvious. Many autistic people have heard, and often intensely dislike, the phrase "you don't look autistic," as if autism has a "look." Usually, Level 1 autistic people have more neurotypical-looking features that make their challenges more confusing to outsiders. Teachers can sometimes see a talented young child recite whole passages of books that interest them, and then be unable to reconcile that same child getting into fights because they make social mistakes no neurotypical peer would. The confusion comes from not knowing that intelligence and social understanding are fundamentally different, although seen as connected because of what society expects of people at certain ages.

What frustrates many autistic people is that it is especially rare to have a person in their life who can see the world from their point of view. It is not an uncommon story for teachers, family, peers, professionals, and later workplace peers and managers to constantly misunderstand an autistic person and lose patience with them. There's another way of looking at this.

As speech-language pathologist and Brown University adjunct professor Barry Prizant titled his 2016 book, autistic people are just "uniquely human." This refers to their ability to learn skills and mature just like neurotypicals do. The difference is that autistic people have a distinctive "starter brain." They are not pre-wired from birth to interact with the world like neurotypicals, which affects how they interact with others and grow as individuals. "Uniquely human" also refers to the tendency for autistic people to sometimes *seem* alien. However, the motives behind their alien presentation are usually deeply relatable to neurotypicals.

Autistic people want human connection, even if it could be unconventional. Many want friends, family, and romantic relationships; they want to survive and be healthy; and they want to be able to pursue their interests. Trying to achieve this is more difficult, however, given that how their brain works goes against much of what most people expect in social interaction and in life generally. This affects how they can handle the world around them.

While many autistic people will likely never approximate a neurotypical presentation, which is not necessarily a desirable goal, some can appear to meet this. With training and conscious effort, they can socialize effectively with neurotypicals in a typical-appearing way. Yet even for this group, it is often exhausting, not just potentially because of sensory issues in their social environments, but autistic people acquire social skills from experience and conscious teaching.[12] This is a more difficult way to learn, especially given that harsh experiences, like bullying and rejection, can cause trauma and resentment that clouds the ability to interact with others in a healthy way.[13]

This method of learning is also more intellectual and rules-based, which means it is less intuitively fluid. If autistic people appear rigid in their social presentation, it could be because they engage in social interaction the same way most neurotypicals solve math problems: intellectually and through rigid steps. This is sometimes even managed with a prescribed set of social rules they follow.[14]

While these rules can be useful in many situations, trying to apply them at more complicated and nuanced times can lead to social breakdown and confusion. *If a person is known to be autistic, it can be a good idea to ask them what they thought they were doing rather than punish them for doing wrong.* There is a good chance their errors are motivated by ignorance, or at least lack of true understanding or ability to regulate emotions, not by selfishness or malice. This is often talked about in the context of children, but as life becomes more socially complicated, this can be especially true of adults.

As stated before, autistic people are not just a diagnostic category. They do not all know each other and may not get along if they do meet, just the same as neurotypicals. Autistic people differ widely in their challenges, their presentations, and their outlooks on life, just like any other group.

Part of what defines a culture is a sense of shared history. Autistic people have many personal stories with common elements that shape how they view the world, and they also have a collective history that gives insight into their common traits.

The story of autism is still largely unknown to most neurotypicals. But just as any anthropologist or sociologist would look at the history of the group they were studying, it helps to understand where autistic people came from, leading to where they are now, and how it has particularly affected adults, whose stories are even less understood.

## A Summary of a Tumultuous History

Autism has likely always been a part of human societies. Even before official diagnostic times, it has been speculated to exist even in scientists like Henry Cavendish in the eighteenth century and investigations of mentally disabled people in Massachusetts in the nineteenth century.[15] But as an idea in modern medicine, autism has its roots in the early twentieth century. In 1911, Swiss psychologist Eugen Bleuler observed unusual traits he thought looked like schizophrenia (a term Bleuler invented) that were likely autism.

Russian psychologist Grunya Sukhareva also noticed them and, in 1926, used the term "autism" to describe some childhood patients.[16]

But the condition we know today is commonly told through two origin stories: one from the United States and one from Austria, both from the 1940s. The first is about Leo Kanner, a precocious child, who by age eighteen could speak six languages. He was Jewish, born in Austria-Hungary in an area that today is Ukraine, and moved to Germany at twelve. He started his career in a Berlin hospital and later fled to the United States in 1924 to avoid the consequences of German hyperinflation, which started destroying its economy in 1923 and eventually helped lead to the rise of the Nazis. Kanner deeply understood the significant timing of his departure, and he took advantage of his new geographical position, later bringing German Jews into his adopted country, saving them from what would have likely been harsh persecution or extermination.

Keep this in mind when Hans Asperger comes up.

After Kanner worked in pediatrics and psychology in a hospital in Yankton, South Dakota, he got a job at Johns Hopkins University in Baltimore in 1938. That year, he met a five-year-old child named Donald Triplett, the son of a well-off bank-owning family in Forest, Mississippi. Triplett displayed unusual behaviours, like not showing affection while being touched and spinning, which we view today as an autistic self-soothing behaviour.

Kanner eventually discovered eleven similar children between 1938 and 1943 that he then described in his first article on autism, published in the journal *Nervous Child*, identifying what he called "autistic disturbances of affective contact."[17] These clients usually came from upper-middle-class white American families like the Tripletts.[18] This fact likely helped someone like Donald get identified, but even more importantly, it helped him get appropriate care from a trained psychologist like Kanner. After spending a brief time in an institution as a young child, Triplett returned to the family home. He eventually went to community college and worked as an employee at the family bank. Hc passed away in June 2023 at the age of eighty-nine.[19]

Kanner's paper is often cited as the world's first major publicly released article about autism. There was also a second researcher, however, who identified a different kind of autism around the same time as Kanner first found his eleven children. Yet it was only after this researcher died in 1980 that people knew his name — both for the great and dark parts of his legacy.

Hans Asperger was an Austrian physician who ran Heilpädagogik Station, a children's clinic in Vienna, where he identified 200 children, many of whom would have likely been referred to by a condition later named after him.[20] Asperger published 300 scientific journal articles in his lifetime, mostly on the topic of what he called "autistic psychopathy."[21] It should be noted that at this time, "psychopathy" meant something more like "personality disorder," rather than the manipulative, conscienceless person the term often refers to today.[22]

In 1944, his first paper was published in German, detailing four of these children with "autistic psychopathy" and summarizing broad aspects of this condition. While some of the language he used to describe the children is harsh by today's standards, the article is remarkable for a person of his time in terms of how much he tried to truly understand his children. He sees them as more than their disability aspects, possibly because he may have had some of these traits as a child and related to them.[23]

Asperger connected what he was seeing in his kids to Bleuler and distinguished "autistic psychopathy" from schizophrenia.[24] He saw their inherent gifts as well as their challenges, even going as far as calling them "little professors." He believed autism was "polygenetic," meaning caused by multiple genes. All these ideas ended up being correct within a model of what it is to be autistic, and with his other ideas, created a foundation for future models.

For decades, it was believed that Kanner and Asperger made these discoveries independent of each other. But it was later revealed in 2015 by journalist Steve Silberman that there was a connection between Kanner and Asperger that helped fuel the discovery.

George Frankl, who had worked with Asperger in Vienna, fled to the United States in 1937 and later worked with Kanner.[25] He is explicitly credited in Kanner's 1943 paper with contributing to this work.[26] What Frankl had seen in Vienna likely influenced the first publication about autism in the United States.

Despite the insight of Asperger, substantial controversy always surrounded the man himself. During his lifetime, Kanner generally downplayed Asperger's achievements and writings, with the reason believed to be that, as a Jewish refugee from Germany, he was suspicious of Asperger's connection to the Nazis in Austria.[27] This suspicion later turned out to have merit.

The degree of Asperger's connection to the Nazis is disputed. His defenders pointed out that he was never a member of the Nazi Party and made speeches to Nazi Party members supportive of treating special needs children with kindness and recognizing their gifts.[28] They also point out he would have been under considerable pressure, including threats to his life, to conform to what Nazi occupiers asked of him.[29] However, there were other aspects of his life — including that his clinic was allowed to operate throughout the war, indicating some level of cooperation with the authorities — that have often raised questions about him. A presentation by Herwig Czech in 2010 and particularly a paper by him in 2018 revealed documentary evidence that Asperger signed off on children from his clinic being sent to the infamous Am Spiegelgrund clinic in Vienna.[30] There, 789 children were killed, and thousands of others were subjected to unethical and cruel experiments by Nazi officials.[31]

Despite what Asperger got right about autism, perhaps before anyone else, his cooperation with the Nazis has significantly marked his legacy. The historical circumstances of his work also meant that it was not widely known for decades, leaving Kanner's model as the predominant way to look at autism. This accident of history revealed the full scope of the Kannerian model's strengths and weaknesses.

## Slow Change

Despite Kanner's heroism in the face of Nazism, he made several important mistakes regarding autism that Asperger never did. The first was about what constituted autism, which affects how prevalent it is thought to be. Autism was considered a rare and obviously spottable condition under Kanner's idea of autism, estimated at about 1 in 5,000 people as late as the 1960s and 1970s.[32] To put this in perspective, Temple Grandin had to take a test for Kannerian autism when she was a child in the 1950s. On that test, she had to score a twenty to qualify as autistic. She scored a nine.[33] While many children who would be diagnosed today were simply overlooked, many others were still seen as different. Sometimes, they were given a label of childhood schizophrenia. True schizophrenia in children is considered rare today, but it harkens back faultily to Bleuler's earliest observations.[34]

Doctors often recommended that children with these labels get placed in institutions, which were the predominant form of care for autistic children, as well as other people with psychological differences and illnesses, from the nineteenth century to the 1970s. Hundreds of thousands of people were estimated to have been put into dozens of institutions in the United States alone.[35]

Institutions were not often nice places. They separated their residents from society, frequently to the point where even the child's family rarely if ever saw them. In some cases, families of institutionalized loved ones were told to remove pictures of them from family photo albums and never speak of them.[36] This even happened to the British royal family, when two of Queen Elizabeth II's cousins were institutionalized.[37]

There was genuine care for residents of these institutions, and often they were even given work opportunities, but mistreatment by staff was also not uncommon, including food neglect and electroshock punishments.[38]

The nature of these institutions resulted in campaigns to deinstitutionalize in the late 1960s. One of the core arguments was that increases in quality psychiatric drugs as well as cheaper and more humane therapies and treatments were better solutions than institutions. The idea that people with disabilities should be integrated into the community has also since become mainstream.

Around this time, the first disability rights movements were emerging, for both physical and neurological conditions. The earliest social models of disability started to gain traction, where disability was seen as something that society imposes on some people rather than something wrong with a person with a disability. Also at this time, autism began to be questioned, like many ideas and institutions in the 1960s and 1970s.

The post-institutional period was filled with an increased interest in autism. The two earliest editions of the *Diagnostic and Statistical Manual*, in 1952 and 1968, which did not include autism, were created while heavily influenced by psychoanalysis, a school of psychology that Sigmund Freud made famous.[39]

Psychoanalysis holds that psychological dysfunction is caused by issues in the unconscious mind, often from childhood. As was common in the 1950s and 1960s, Kanner attributed autism to cold and distant parenting in early childhood, which was based on psychoanalytic theory.[40] This was also attributed to the fact he saw many cases among upper-middle-class children and subjectively perceived a certain type of mother in these families. He ended up being wrong about the profile and about the mothers. Because it was largely women who took care of children during this period, coldness on the part of the mother became the common factor associated with the cause of autism. This theory later became popularized through the work of Bruno Bettelheim, who despite his personal advertisements, had questionable (at best) credentials as a psychologist.[41] His 1967 book, *The Empty Fortress*, used the term "refrigerator mother," which stuck.

While even Kanner himself later expressed regret for helping to spread this idea, rebellion against it first came through many parents, most notably Bernie Rimland, who had an autistic son.[42] He wrote a book called *Infantile Autism*, rejecting the refrigerator mother theory and, along with Ruth Sullivan and Ivar Lovaas, formed the National Society of Autistic Children in 1965.[43] It is now the Autism Society of America, whose name crucially implies the existence of autistic adults.

Other organizations, such as the National Autistic Society in England (founded 1962) and the Autism Society of Canada (founded 1976, later merged in 2015 into Autism Canada), were also founded around this time. They became the foundation of a move from an odd clinical interest to a real civil rights movement led by parents, at least for now.

On top of changes in how parents viewed autism, academic models also started to change. During this period, theoretical cognitive models of childhood autism emerged through the partnership of Beate Hermelin and Neil O'Connor, who looked to understand how the autistic mind worked rather than assume it was defective.[44] But these models also resulted from practical analysis and application starting to play a part in very early research about autistic adults.

One of the first studies on autistic adults was conducted by Kanner himself, as he followed up with his original eleven children as adults in 1971. This was a very early attempt to do research on autistic adults, after what he called an "explosion" of new research building on autism in general; what was then considered Kanner's legacy.

Kanner found that two of the original children, Donald Triplett and Frederick W., were "real success stories" by his estimation. He defined "success" roughly as holding a job, being able to pursue their interests, and having lives that are meaningfully connected and where they can make decisions for themselves. Four of the children, who were institutionalized for most of their lives, "lost their luster," according to Kanner, perhaps to some degree foreshadowing the fate of such institutions, which by then were just starting to go into decline. Three of these children who were not in institutions were mildly functional, including one who ended up on a farm doing "functions of a kind, helpful, competent orderly." One of his other children died at age twenty-nine.[45]

In 1973, Kanner wrote a second follow-up on autistic adults, surveying ninety-six of his childhood patients to determine their life circumstances. The overwhelming majority were still living with their parents and not living independent lives.[46]

Ways of figuring out how to help autistic children were starting to emerge around the same time. One of the most enduring attempts to do this was by Eric Schopler and Robert Reichler, who worked out of the University of North Carolina at Chapel Hill. They are most famous today as the founders of Treatment and Education of Autistic and related Communications Handicapped Children (TEACCH), which was first implemented in a North Carolina statewide program in 1972. TEACCH is an education and support program based on visual-information processing, rather than text, and highly structured schedules for autistic children. These ideas inspired later popular education models and remain influential in the care of autistic people, including adults, whom TEACCH still serves to this day.[47]

This development also reflects a division in psychology that started to emerge at this time. Ivar Lovaas, one of the founders of the National Society of Autistic Children, also applied (but did not discover despite common misconception) the therapeutic principles of applied behavioural analysis (ABA). This application, which began in the 1960s and exploded in popularity in the 1980s,[48] started one of the main ideological debates in the world of autism.

Schopler and Lovaas disliked each other personally and because they represented two conflicting theories of psychology relating to autism.[49] Schopler was at the forefront of developmental psychology, which looks at how a person's thinking, and personality changes throughout their life, affects their decisions and influences their engagement with people on that level. At the core of TEACCH is the attempt to structure a program that considers what a person's mindset is.

In the autistic context, developmental psychologists would ask these kinds of questions:

- How do autistic people see the world?
- Are autistic people more likely to be productive if their work is done by a schedule that they are comfortable with?
- Are they more likely to be productive if they are interested?

In contrast, Lovaas represented behaviourism, which comes from B.F. Skinner's theories in the 1950s, that says human behaviour is affected primarily by consequences. If there are positive consequences, the behaviour will be more likely to happen again. If there are negative consequences, the behaviour will be less likely to happen. This is the foundation of ABA, and ABA-based therapies are still widely used, with a large body of evidence showing that it successfully teaches functioning and social skills to autistic people.[50]

However, the self-advocacy community now tends to view ABA with hostility. It is a highly contentious topic. While it will come up later in this book because it is so essential to understanding a lot about the world of autism today, an answer to whether ABA is beneficial is well beyond the scope of this book.

In the 1960s and 1970s, there were more studies searching for causes of autism. British psychologist Michael Rutter was particularly influential, especially with his twin study in 1977, which found that if one identical twin was autistic, up to 60% of the time the other was also.[51] When these studies were conducted under subsequent changes to autism criteria, they raised this estimate to 90%.[52]

Studies such as these went a long way in disproving the "refrigerator mother" hypothesis. Autism largely comes from genes but is also mixed with currently unknown environmental factors, not cold parenting. But the recognition of autism as a condition with true society-wide implications was just beginning.

## A New Way of Seeing Autism

The momentum of greater activism, recognition, and research carried on until 1980, when autism was added to the DSM for the first time. This DSM-III edition was the first that tried to move away from the psychoanalytic model and into a more practical and scientific model. This DSM was not just a game changer in autism, it was also a bestseller.[53]

Spurred by the inclusion of autism in the DSM, the 1980s also brought a new wave of research about autism. In 1983, one study produced the first major work published on autistic adults, *Autism in Adults and Adolescents*, by Eric Schopler and Gary Mesibov, at the University of North Carolina at Chapel Hill, featuring contributions from many of the leading autism researchers at the time. In the 1980s, such a book was revelatory. This was the first real attempt by prominent experts to try and publish something significant about autistic adults, who were not just becoming understood but recognized as even existing.

Schopler's introduction, "Can an Adolescent or Adult Have Autism?," is typical of the level of debate that existed up to this time, as he wrote: "When that question was asked one or two decades ago, most people familiar with 'autism' would have said 'Certainly not.'"[54]

Among the contributors to this book was Lorna Wing, who by then was already starting to revolutionize the field of autism. A researcher in England, she made four important and connected discoveries around this time which contributed to this achievement.

- She conducted a study in the London suburb of Camberwell with her research partner, Judith Gould, which was published in 1979. There, they completed a census and determined that the prevalence of autism by Kannerian standards was accurate, but that many people with autistic traits did not strictly meet the Kannerian profile.

- She discovered and translated Hans Asperger's work, with the help of her German-speaking husband, John Wing. This included Asperger's famous 1944 paper. She published her own paper coining the term "Asperger's syndrome" in 1981.
- She originated the idea of the triad of impairments in autistic people — issues with "social imagination," "social interaction," and "repetitive behaviours" — which later formed the core of clinical diagnosis in later editions of the DSM.
- She coined the term "autism spectrum" to reconcile Kanner and Asperger's discoveries.[55]

This broadening of the autism spectrum led to many autistic people who had not been recognized previously getting a diagnosis. Pervasive developmental disorder-not otherwise specified (PDD-NOS), an outlier form of autism that exists when other autism categories do not match with a person's presentation, was added to an amended DSM-III in 1987. Asperger's syndrome, which was called Asperger's disorder, was added to the DSM-IV in 1994, a diagnoses that broadly reflected Hans Asperger's "little professor." This expansion of the criteria for having an autistic condition produced an explosion of diagnosis in the 1990s. Coupled with greater public awareness through moments like the release of the 1988 movie *Rain Man*, this also led to increased community activism and attention from lawmakers.[56]

The era of the expansion of diagnoses, roughly from 1981 to 1995, also led to several new developments. The first coincided with the move towards deinstitutionalization, which was already fairly well-advanced. As institutions were starting to fall out of favour, there was a lot of interest in how autistic adults should live in a post-institutional setting.

Norman and Jane Giddon's *Autistic Adults at Bittersweet Farms*, published in 1991, promoted a rural residential care model that was attempted at Bittersweet Farms in northwest Ohio. In other places, including Canada, facilities like Silver Spring Farm in Ottawa tried to do something similar.[57] Autistic people would live in a farm-type lodging at a large garden, do chores, learn communication skills, and have communal meals.[58] "Going out in the community" was the key aspect these places hoped to emphasize, since people who ran them were keen to stress that their residents were not hidden from society as in prior facilities.[59] Institutions where autistic people went out into the community were seen as progressive and reflecting real change. In retrospect, though, while Bittersweet Farms is still active and studies show its model has benefits, places like it have not been widely replicated.[60] This may be in part because they require a lot of space and therefore are difficult to scale to the number of individuals who need them. The problem of assisted care for autistic adults, especially after their parents can no longer provide care, is still a major unsolved issue in North American society.

The second development of this era of activism was in education. This led directly to the United States government passing the Americans with Disabilities Act in 1990 and the Individuals with Disabilities in Education Act (IDEA) the same year, which provided coverage up to the age of twenty-one and ensured equal access to education with individual accommodations. It also updated the Education for Handicapped Children Act from 1975, which legislated equal access to education but did not lay out rules for individual accommodations like IDEA did.[61]

It was also during this time that Canadian provinces started bringing in their first autism support programs, which will be looked at in more detail in part 2.

The third development was that autistic adults themselves spoke out in the popular press for the first time. Temple Grandin's first book, *Emergence: Labeled Autistic*, was published in 1986, and made her internationally famous. Bernie Rimland called it "the first book written by a recovered autistic individual" (he was right that Grandin's text was a pioneering work, but wrong about her being "recovered").[62] Grandin's perspective was and remains autobiographical and practical. Her writing often uses standard technical language about autism and features practical advice to both autistic people and parents, often from her own experience but also through citing academic literature. This approach has often been seen in contrast to another one, which preferred to look at society's view of how disabled people are treated. This has become perhaps the main distinction of views from within the autistic community.

In 1993, Jim Sinclair, a non-binary person who goes by the pronoun "xe," wrote "Don't Mourn for Us," an essay that became the basis of the self-advocacy movement.[63] It included this famous passage, summing up the attitudes many autistic people now wanted to fight: "When parents say, I wish my child did not have autism, what they're really saying is, I wish the autistic child I have did not exist, and I had a different (non-autistic) child instead."[64]

This summed up how many autistic people, including by now many adults, felt about their condition. Autism is a condition with challenges, but also real benefits. Many autistic people do not experience their condition as something that causes suffering. It helps them form their identity, and it is something they wish to assert that they are proud to have.

Whereas Grandin's approach was more about improving autistic people's lives through helping them adapt to the neurotypical world, Sinclair's view placed much emphasis on autistic self-respect and assertion of one's identity, as well as focus on societal and systemic barriers. Like the debate between the autistic and autism communities, this is not necessarily a binary. Whether someone emphasizes one over the other does have certain ideological connotations within the autism world. This is a major dividing line, even sometimes among autistic people.

The broader research community started to catch on to adults a bit later, in the late 1990s and early 2000s. In 1997, Patricia Howlin published *Autism and Asperger Syndrome: Preparing for Adulthood*. In her 2004 edition, Howlin said that, during the years in between editions, there was an "explosion" of interest in adults.[65]

There were likely many reasons why this occurred. The first is that the initial wave of children diagnosed in the late '80s and early '90s were coming into adolescence and adulthood. This meant the complexion of diagnosed autistic adults changed from a generally rare, more obvious expression to a wide range of individuals that many people would likely encounter in their lives. This range of expression applied to those with classic Kannerian traits and those who work in Silicon Valley.

This was also reflected more in the popular press. Among the most famous articles was one by Steve Silberman, a journalist for *WIRED*, who wrote "The Geek Syndrome" in 2001, which looked at autism in the world of Silicon Valley.[66] This article became a major success whose reception inspired Silberman to publish *Neurotribes* in 2015, which was about the history of autism and the neurodiversity movement and won him the then-called Samuel Johnson Prize.[67]

There was also a further increase in fiction about autism. Movies like 2001's *I Am Sam*, about a more obviously presenting autistic father played by Sean Penn, and *The Curious Incident of the Dog in the Night-Time*, a 2003 Mark Haddon book about an imaginative, less obviously autistic graduating high-school student, came out and put the broader autism spectrum into more public consciousness.

Academic studies also continued to increase throughout the rest of the

2000s. A PubMed search showed cited articles on "autism adults" going up from 246 in 2005 to 624 in 2010.[68]

But while research, public interest, and diagnoses were exploding, there was also still a highly active parent and research movement throughout the 1990s and 2000s. These organizations had a lot of public influence and held a variety of different views. More common at the time was that they saw autism as a pathology that had to be treated, and in some cases needed to be cured.

This expressed itself in two influential ways. One came in the form of genetics research, such as through Jonathan Shestack's organization Cure Autism Now that used a large genetic collection in an attempt to find a cure.[69] It was later absorbed into Autism Speaks in 2007, an organization founded by General Electric vice-chairman Bob Wright and his wife, Suzanne, in 2005, after the diagnosis of their autistic grandson.[70] This is the largest, and most controversial, autism organization in the world today, described as a "behemoth" in an autism community that has always been contentious and full of competing organizations.[71]

Proponents of the organization have praised its fundraising ability and reach and, therefore, its ability to bring awareness to autism. Its blue puzzle piece logo, which is the most famous symbol of autism, has become synonymous with autism itself and the Autism Speaks organization, reflective of its marketing power.

It is also essential to note that the organization is controversial enough that even displaying its symbols can spark passionate anger among its critics.[72] It has been strongly criticized, particularly by self-advocates, for the way it spends its money, specifically in prioritizing research into the causes of autism over funding services.[73] It has also been denounced for its lack of hiring autistic people,[74] its perceived pathologizing of autism,[75] and its historic endorsement of a cure, which they rejected in 2016.[76]

The second influential development was more inflammatory, more unhinged, and yet even more influential on the discussion of autism than the first. In 1998, Andrew Wakefield, a now decertified doctor from England, published a study in the prestigious medical journal *The Lancet* claiming that the measles, mumps, and rubella vaccine (known as MMR vaccine) caused autism.[77] The study was later shown to be fraudulent, but it had triggered a large movement against vaccines in general, which included celebrities like Jenny McCarthy and even some autism activists like Bernie

Rimland.[78] It sparked a hearing specifically dedicated to the subject in the U.S. Congress in 2002.[79]

Many autistic people saw not just a scientific issue with the movement but also saw the anti-vaccine movement as an attack on *them*. If parents were not getting their children vaccinated because of fears of autism, it implied that they believed autism was worse than measles, mumps, rubella, and possibly many other preventable diseases. There was also a much less subjective and more fundamental problem. In the intervening years, a large body of evidence emerged that showed no link between vaccines and autism. In 2010, Wakefield was stripped of his medical license.[80]

The vaccine hypothesis was also tolerated, if not endorsed, by major autism organizations. Autism Speaks did not take a position against the vaccine hypothesis publicly until 2015.[81] But while much of the autism and autistic communities were fixated on this issue, other important developments were happening.

## Building on Wing

By the time the DSM-5 came out in 2013, the consensus of psychologists had become more like Lorna Wing's idea of an autism spectrum, rather than the cluster of diagnoses in the DSM-IV. The eleventh edition of the *International Classification of Diseases*, released in 2022, also introduced the autism spectrum to European clinicians who use this book to guide diagnosis instead of the DSM.[82]

The view that was becoming more accepted by autism experts around the time the DSM-5 was being discussed was that of the British clinician Tony Attwood, one of the leading autism experts in the world. He weighed in publicly on the difference between Asperger's syndrome and what was called "high-functioning autism," a term that, like Wing's use of Asperger's syndrome, was first described in 1981: "As a clinician, I do not think that academics should try to force a dichotomy when the profiles of social and behavioural abilities are so similar, and the treatment is the same."[83]

At the time, this was controversial, particularly because many autistic people embraced their DSM-IV labels. Asperger's syndrome diagnosis holders, who sometimes referred to themselves as Aspies, particularly had an attachment to their label.

There was also the more practical concern that, while one of the supporting arguments was that an autism label would fit more readily into government programs, autistic people feared losing their old diagnostic labels and, therefore, becoming ineligible for services.

Michael John Carley is an autistic self-advocate who founded the Global and Regional Asperger's Syndrome Partnership (GRASP), later changed to Global and Regional Autism Spectrum Partnership in 2003, which became known in autism circles for its support groups for autistic people. He was one of the early opponents of this change for precisely this reason. While not opposed to Lorna Wing's autism spectrum idea per se, he believed a change would create a problem bureaucratically that could make life harder for autistic people. "I did change my mind about this," he said. "I changed my mind only after I found out that people would, despite the DSM committee's promises, lose their diagnoses."

People like Carley and researchers in favour of the change ended up being right. There was a greater chance that a professional diagnosis of autism would match a service provider's criteria for autism, making it more likely that an autistic person qualified for services.

There were some people on the spectrum, however, that may not qualify under the new diagnosis, particularly older adults, girls, and those with fewer obvious traits, who may have fallen under a diagnosis like Asperger's but not strictly meet a new diagnosis.[84]

What all this shows is that, even if the diagnostic manuals were right scientifically, the changes could cause problems bureaucratically, which is always a consideration with the DSM and ICD. This also shows the greater complexity of dealing with autism as an issue. This is where the DSM is at today, but it is not where the inquiry ended.

In 2014, a group of writers led by Fred Volkmar, the head of the Yale Child Study Center, published *Adolescents and Adults with Autism Spectrum Disorders*. The work is specifically dedicated to Schopler, who died in 2006, and Mesibov, who as of this writing is still alive. But Volkmar and his colleagues had more than thirty years of extra knowledge to build on for their book.

The first obvious clue of difference is in the titles: autism vs. autism *spectrum*. This change reflects the changes in attitude and understanding of autism from Schopler to the last decade, both reflecting the acceptance of Wing's ideas and seeing autism encompassing a fuller range of people.

As the authors explicitly note, the approach to studying autism has also dramatically changed:

> In 1983, Schopler and Mesibov's earlier book on this topic addressed topics relevant to adults, such as education, medical care, behavior problems, sexuality, family issues, and independent living. At that time, most knowledge was based on case reports, clinical experience, anecdote, and occasional open intervention studies.[85]

The last decade has also produced a much larger number of texts dedicated to autistic adults. Multiple other academic compendiums have also been published, such as *Autism Spectrum Disorders in Adults* (2017) by Bernardo Barahona-Correa and Rutger-Jan van der Gaag, and *Autism in Adulthood* (2019) by Susan Lowinger and Shiri Pearlman-Avnion, which has a disproportionate focus on Israeli adults and the role of the Israeli Defence Forces in forming the identity of adults.

The hope among academics is that more autism journals and compendiums like these will be released based on high-quality research. Although there has been a relatively quick increase in the last ten years, Volkmar acknowledges there is still a long way to go: "In the three decades that have elapsed since its [Schopler and Mesibov's book] publication, methods and the overall volume of research in ASD have dramatically improved, but adolescence and adulthood in ASD remain rather poorly understood."[86]

Despite nearly a decade passing since it was published, this sentence could be written today. By comparison to autism's past, this problem seems refreshingly solvable. After eugenics, institutionalization, misdiagnosis, confusion, stigma, rediscovery, and now self-assertion, autistic people progressed from a totally unrecognized entity to a major disability community and a visible and formidable group in society.

The net result today is a situation and awareness of autism that is better than it ever has been, but not without getting a lot wrong in the past and not without many lingering problems. Among these include a disconnect between parents, researchers, and autistic people themselves; a diagnosis that can be life-changing but also spark as many questions as answers; and a confusing patchwork of programs and services that are hard to navigate and make it even harder for autistic people to get what they need. That means a compromised quality of life among autistic people themselves.

Then there is another complicating factor, which is age. As shown throughout much of the history of autism, the focus was on kids. Only comparatively recently is the reality taken seriously that those same kids grow up.

## CHAPTER 2:
# AUTISTIC ADULTS TODAY

Autistic people went from non-existent in 1940, to rare in 1970, to now an estimated one in forty-four people in the United States.[1] This proportion is similar to the size of the LGBTQ+, Jewish, or Muslim populations in North America.[2]

This number has also gone up dramatically over the last forty years. In the 1980s, only one in thousands of people were diagnosed. In the 1990s, it was one in hundreds. In 2000, it was one in 150, and in 2008, it was one in eighty-eight.[3] This increase has affected rates in society as a whole, though there are some groups in Western countries, especially women, ethnic minorities, and those with less obvious traits, who are thought to be underdiagnosed.

The real number of autistic people is still unknown. One major Yale University study in South Korea determined the number of autistic people there to be one in thirty-eight, but this is still just an estimate.[4]

What is even more important is that the percentage of autistic adults compared to neurotypical adults is believed to be roughly the same as the number of autistic children compared to neurotypical children.[5] Because there are more adults than children, this means there are more autistic adults in the world than autistic children. Therefore, it becomes useful to talk about autism in a different way than the traditional child-centred approach, which has been the focus throughout much of the modern history of autism.

Autistic adults have different issues from autistic children, so much so that it challenges how autism is viewed as a whole. In the clinical community, autism is often looked at as a series of cognitive differences, challenges, and behaviours because in children this is how they are perceived by outsiders.

There is some attention to seeing positive traits of autistic people too, but there's an innocence in much of this analysis that can overlook complicating factors that emerge over the course of a person's life.

When many people look at an autistic person, they often ask "why do they have these traits?" but they do not ask "what has their life been like?" This is where autistic adults can fill the gaps because there has been time to answer that question in their lives, by definition.

Autism isn't usually viewed by the public through the lens of factors like trauma, which is less comfortable to think about than innate brain structures. When thinking about autism and development, images of children lining up blocks are more comforting than autistic adults alone in their bedrooms ruminating about the neglect and abuse that may have occurred throughout their life.

Autism is also not often looked at through the lens of historically taboo topics like sex, in both its positive and negative manifestations. It is also not looked at through factors like repeated social and familial stigma or mental illness.

Looking at autism through the lens of childhood can give a sense that autistic people are pure and innocent, even though autistic people have all the frailties and potential of neurotypicals. In other words, they have all the things that make people and life interesting.

Let's look at autistic adults through a series of questions. The first one is: *Who are autistic adults as a group today?*

The answer is it really depends on the person, but there are some trends. The autistic adult community is made up of men, women, and a disproportionately high number of people who don't identify as either. This could be people who identify as the opposite of their biological gender or or as non-binary.

The autistic adult community comprises people of all cultures and socioeconomic backgrounds, though a disproportionate number of autistic adults are unemployed, underemployed, or struggle economically. It also includes people with various different presentations, from some with intellectual disabilities to others with genius-level IQs, from individuals who live largely free of support to others who need a lot of outside support.

Autistic adults also appear differently to outsiders. One person can be barely recognizable to an outsider as autistic. Another may be immediately recognizably autistic, or at least different, to someone who is unfamiliar with autism. This presentation is based on traits naturally present from birth as well as the person's early development and support throughout life. Their traits can be more noticeable on different days and in various settings, whether it is at home, school, or work. It may also be dependent on what is going on in their life and environment. More stress in their life might mean more obvious signs, for example.

Autism does not get more obvious over time on its own, but an unsupportive environment can make autistic people more prone to negative outcomes over time.[6] This is relevant for autistic people as a group as they are more likely to endure more "adverse childhood experiences" than the general population, meaning that by adulthood they are more likely to have been neglected or physically abused by caregivers.[7] This makes them statistically more prone to struggle with physical and mental health issues.

By adulthood, some autistic people have sufficient learned skills and adaptive abilities that help them adjust in the world. A small percentage even learn enough that they do not fall into a clinical diagnosis of autism.[8] This does not mean these people cease to be autistic, but the hindrance autism has on their lives no longer requires consistent clinical monitoring. This is not the majority, however.

In addition to those currently recognized as clinically autistic, who are the focus of this book, the idea of a "broader autism phenotype" currently exists within the psychiatric community. This is an extension of the autism spectrum that even includes people who present some traits of autism but who do not quite qualify for a clinical diagnosis.[9] Rates of autism among people with this broad phenotype vary widely from study to study, and it is not yet as well-defined as traditional clinically diagnosable autism.[10]

Many if not most autistic and non-autistic people see autism as a disability, at least in part. Its traits can be traceable to aspects of a person's life that make it difficult to hold a job, carry out day-to-day tasks, and lead an independent life, making them likely to rely on disability benefits.

But they also see something else. As will be covered in much more detail throughout this book, the sensory issues, perhaps with noise, which can limit the number of jobs an autistic person could comfortably hold, are also the same issues that can lead to remarkable talents in something like music. Isolation can reflect an autistic person's loneliness, or it can be necessary for an autistic person to hyperfocus and do remarkable work.

Autistic traits are often extreme versions of what all people experience. Also, like everyone else, the ability for autistic people to discover and understand themselves is frequently what can make the difference between how well they can manage life.

This gets to the second question. *How do autistic adults perceive their experiences?*

This answer also depends on the individual, but there are trends as well as broader societal factors that play into it. The comparative lack of research on autistic adults has meant that, until very recently, clinicians did not have much verifiable evidence to measure their experience. Even today, there is still a shortage of extensive long-term studies of autistic adults. For some adult groups, like those over forty, the lack of literature in general persists. While this is changing, and there are great resources for autistic adults, the overall lack of research has meant a lack of effective services because most serious service providers understandably like to base what they provide on evidence.

Even more importantly, it is difficult for autistic adults to truly understand themselves. If society broadly understands how healthy neurotypical children develop but not how healthy autistic children develop, there are no models and reasonable expectations for how autistic adults can grow to be their best.

Autistic adults often compare themselves to their neurotypical peers, perhaps because there is no real alternative. Because autistic people can really do well in some areas and struggle in others, this can sometimes create unrealistic expectations from other people and themselves for what they can do. For example, if an autistic person has learned to socialize to the point that they're not seen as obviously autistic, why do they have issues with a little noise at an office party?

Without a healthier and more realistic way of seeing themselves in society, autistic adults can be left feeling depressed. This is where a strictly clinical understanding of autism can often fall short of encapsulating the experience of being autistic. Autistic adults do not see their own experiences through a collection of symptoms or through broad trends, as useful as this can be in many contexts. Before they are diagnosed, autistic adults did not see themselves as disabled the same way a person in a wheelchair understands that their legs or muscles don't work, yet they often knew something was different about them from childhood. This is one of the elusive aspects of an invisible condition. For many people, especially those who could not get a diagnosis, this was often a confusing, frustrating, and even existential experience.

These frustrations and challenges can lead to trauma. Like any other person, individuals deal with this in their own ways. Some bury their traumas, don't think too much about their autism, and try to carry on with their lives. Some autistic people have difficulties taking care of themselves, and others can perceive this lack of independence in many ways.

Other autistic people form communities with people who have the same diagnosis, some of which make their communities political action organizations. Like any community, these efforts can produce healthy experiences based on positive ways of dealing with a shared experience, or unhealthy experiences based on resentment.

While encountering a neurotypical world is difficult and sometimes even traumatic, there are also advantages and even great gifts associated with autism. The tendency towards solitude and a fascination with personal interests, which is characteristic of a disproportionately high number of autistic people, can be a great advantage in career-related pursuits and can give meaning to their private life. Other common personality aspects of autism also have advantages, such as honesty and reliability, a strong sense of justice, and a comparative lack of prejudice. A person with a strong moral code that is difficult to break can seem naïve and frustrating if the person is misguided, but strong principles are usually celebrated in a person who knows who they are and has a strong conscience.

These strong personality aspects often complicate the views of many autistic adults. Autistic brains themselves are not defective and do not cause harm to those who have them. This lack of direct harm that comes from autism, coupled with the benefits it can bring, form the basis of the idea of neurodiversity. Since these brains also provide joy and satisfaction to the person and others, it should be thought of as a different cognitive style rather than a defect.

This way of thinking leads to questions about how autistic people can be recognized and understood for both their gifts *and* challenges. Broader neurotypical society may not always consider the presence and value of autistic people. This is not a harsh moral judgment of this society as many people do not consciously meet autistic people in their daily lives and are not forced to think about these questions. However, this is an acknowledgment of the need for popular understanding to catch up because being perceived as having value in society means a lot to autistic people.

An essential place to start with this perception is to help neurotypicals recognize when a person may have autistic traits.

## How to Identify and Relate to Autistic Adults

Most people in Western societies today at some level recognize the need to treat people with disabilities, including autism, with appropriate basic respect. But unlike many disabilities, such as being paraplegic or having Down syndrome, there are not always obvious physical markers with autism, which can complicate how a neurotypical initially perceives an autistic person.

It has been recognized even since Kanner that autism does not have a "look."[11] The question then is, in real life, how does someone recognize that another person may be autistic?

There are two problems. One: Ordinary people cannot and should not try to be amateur diagnosticians. Only a trained professional who has done a clinical and ethical assessment should attempt to diagnose an autistic person. The following information is more detailed in chapters 3 and 4 and offers only general guidelines to identify if a person *might* be autistic.

Two: Autism is highly variable, a major reason why autism can present in so many ways. Genetic research suggests autism can be expressed in as many as 1,000 different genes, with many possible environmental causes contributing to whether someone is autistic.[12] These range from the father's age to the environment in the mother's womb.

Making this even more complicated is that autistic adults can learn coping mechanisms to conceal their traits. People can look less autistic in a diagnostic interview than they are in real life, which can even lead to misdiagnosis.[13] They can seem less autistic in their workplace than at home because they may talk more readily there, or they may have more energy at the start of the day than the end. Some autistic people learn to conceal certain interests and mimic neurotypical social behaviours, which they do at work but not with a group of autistic people, for example.

Regardless of the potential problems, identifying possible autism traits in an individual is useful because this can help others to treat them appropriately. If someone makes a social mistake, and another person understands they even *might* be autistic, the mistake may be viewed differently than if the person is presumed to just be rude. If most similar scenarios are treated with understanding, this makes a significant difference in the life of an autistic person.

Finding these clues is also critical because it is far from a guarantee that an autistic person would feel comfortable saying whether they are autistic or not, and some neurotypicals may not feel comfortable asking.

In some autistic people, identifying their traits can be relatively easy. There can be non-speaking or grunting. They could be constantly echoing movie lines or video games while not responding to people talking about other topics. They could be screaming while covering their ears at a grocery store from overstimulation. They may be showing obvious self-soothing mechanisms, called "stims", that non-autistic people almost never use, like rocking violently back and forth. These expressions of autism are more obvious and easily recognizable to most people as indicating someone who is different. While someone grunting audibly in a grocery store can attract unwanted attention, it may result in others having immediate understanding and empathy for them.

These people are more often diagnosed because such challenges need the kind of support that's not readily available except through diagnosis. Therefore, those who are around autistic people are more likely to have a coherent and readily understood explanation for their presentation should it cause embarrassment or problems.

The struggles of less obviously autistic people are also significant, even if they are not intellectually disabled and do everyday tasks that a more obviously autistic person struggles with.

Sometimes autism can be evident when a conversation starts. They may not make eye contact, they may fidget, they may be stiff, they can be distractible, or they may stay silent, doing so because they really must take time to process what someone is saying. They may also talk a lot about a particular subject of interest, they may stand too close to the other person, or they may notice little patterns that completely escape the other's notice.

Sometimes they only reveal these traits when they are in areas of weakness. These can include sensory issues, such as if they are in a place with bright lights, a noisy situation like a fire drill, or an unfamiliar restaurant with food they don't like. They may also have triggers, such as people shouting, that make them more prone to extreme emotional reactions.

In themselves, none of these are tell-tale signs of autism, of course, but they all indicate that autism *may* be there. Even if these traits are present and autism is not the reason, they should be treated with appropriate respect and should not be stigmatized. *If someone is struggling socially, give that person space. If a person needs to take extra time to respond to someone, whether they are autistic or not, this should be given without judgment.*

This is often more difficult for many people than it sounds. Human beings are prone to picking up even minor signs of difference, and sometimes this is treated with hostility. *If what a person is doing is not directly hurting someone, it is often best to take the time to understand them rather than treat them as a problem to be solved or, even worse, as a threat.* Handling the difference with understanding makes an enormous impact in an autistic adult's life.

However, part of the struggle of autistic people with less obvious traits, who are a large percentage, is convincing others and sometimes even themselves that they have challenges. As King's College London professor and globally famous autism researcher Patricia Howlin says, "society in general also tends to be less sympathetic of individuals whose needs or disabilities are relatively mild . . . expectations are often unrealistically high."[14]

Less obviously autistic people can be baffling to others because they may do remarkable things while sometimes challenged with basic self-care and social interaction. When they make a social mistake, they can sometimes be labelled as difficult, rude, or unpleasant, whereas a more obviously autistic person might be recognized for their disability. This leads to intense frustration for the autistic person.

*It is better to assume a social mistake might be a result of something like trauma or disability than intentional malice.* People feel less guilty about mocking or ignoring them because they can justify a less obviously autistic person's behaviour as contemptable and obnoxious, rather than as reflecting a disability.

Therefore, noticing possible autism is not only necessary, but it could also improve the quality of an autistic person's life. This also requires people to see autism differently.

## Other Things to Know

It is important not just to treat an autistic adult with respect but also to understand their virtues. An autistic person can be far stronger and more capable than they may first appear. Statistically speaking, an autistic adult is more likely to have experienced bullying, abuse from family members — including sexual abuse, rejection, isolation — and an upward struggle in employment and dating, which most neurotypicals do not have to undergo. Not all autistic people go through all these things, but they are very likely to endure pain which is less common among neurotypicals. If they are still around, have ambition, and are not nihilistic, this reflects their character as well.

Another way autistic people of all kinds, where obviously presenting, have been most unfairly denigrated is through minimizing their intelligence. While there is intellectual disability in autism, and likely more common than among the general population, its extent is unknown. However, even the most conservative estimates suggest most autistic people are not intellectually disabled.

It can also be more difficult to explain an autistic person's intelligence. In both more and less obviously autistic people, estimating intelligence can be an unusually elusive task. Asperger described one of his earliest patients, a boy he called Fritz V., as someone for whom conventional intelligence tests did not work. The results were, in Asperger's words, "highly contradictory."[15]

This is also evidenced in people's own accounts. Maureen Bennie, who runs the Autism Awareness Centre, has an adult boy and a girl who are conspicuously autistic, though both are speaking and not intellectually disabled. She and her husband decided early on that they loved their children for who they were and would not try to change them because, like with Fritz V., the strengths of autism were as meaningful as the challenges. "We accepted early on that our children had certain personalities," Bennie said. "What was the result of autistic tendencies? We decided that the two things mixed so tightly, how do you separate the two things? I don't necessarily think you can."

There are real and significant challenges involved in raising autistic children, which should not be understated. These can involve parents sacrificing their careers to provide appropriate care, including into adulthood, and dealing with problems that would not exist with neurotypical children. This can include finding a place where adult children will be taken care of when the parents cannot anymore.

Some parents are also not as understanding as Bennie, and the results for autistic people raised by such parents can, therefore, be much worse. However, a joyful relationship between more obviously autistic people and others in their lives can also be strongly present, even if it is sometimes less apparent from the outside.

Bennie admits challenges looking into her now-adult children's futures but is equally willing to acknowledge talents, such as her daughter's aptitude in writing. When there has historically been more of an emphasis on challenges raising autistic people, emphasizing the love and possibilities is especially meaningful and equally worthwhile.

The last way this assumption should be questioned is that, throughout this book, readers will be introduced to challenges that autistic people face every day.

Even the ordinary autistic person, who is not an autistic celebrity like Elon Musk or Anthony Hopkins, manages life in ways that can be noble and even inspiring.[16] These are not limited people, as is so often presumed, but people who often do amazingly well given the challenges they face. These are individuals who should be presumed competent until they show otherwise, not the other way around.

## Conclusion

Over the last century, there has been much greater progress identifying the needs of autistic people, which has led to remarkable gains for them as a group. This is due to a lot of research and activism from parents of autistic people, academics, and autistic people themselves. Even today, however, there are still significant struggles for autistic people, including autistic adults.

The next two chapters will deal with the two universal traits required to be diagnosed as autistic: social skills difficulties and restricted and repetitive behaviours. These chapters aim to give as broad a sense of autistic adults as possible.

The DSM-5 criteria, which they are based on, are meant to aid in clinical assessment and show how these traits affect the autistic person's life. For every challenging aspect reflected in the DSM, there is also another positive side to many of these traits and how they are presented, which can help neurotypicals understand why they do what they do and why it makes sense given how an autistic person's brain works.

There is also the approach of Kevin Stoddart, who runs the Redpath Centre in Toronto, which provides private autism services from a neurodiversity viewpoint. He writes about seeing autistic people's problems as a matter of mutual understanding, which is sometimes under-practiced in clinical settings and is a mindset that is often beneficial when dealing with someone whose perceptions of the world are unlike that of the person giving the service.

At all times, the notion of "client as expert" should be reinforced and a "cross-cultural" therapeutic dialogue nurtured.[17]

This "cross-cultural" idea is a particularly useful concept. The problems with understanding autistic people can be more like those of an American understanding someone who is Japanese, rather than a doctor fixing the problems of a sick person.

This viewpoint will both give a glimpse of the complexities of being autistic and help illuminate the misunderstandings and challenges of a deeply remarkable group of people.

# CHAPTER 3:
# SOCIAL COMMUNICATION

THE DSM-5 LISTS SOCIAL COMMUNICATION and social interaction as its first core criteria for diagnosing autism. The subcategories of this deficit include difficulty holding a conversation, issues with non-verbal communication, and problems forming and maintaining friendships.

Communication difficulties are often deeply frustrating for autistic people, even while the specifics of how these issues present vary among them. These include relying on technology and gestures to communicate, to a long list of differences in how the brain processes and manages verbal conversation.

However, struggles with neurotypical-style communication does not indicate lack of thoughts. It just means it can be difficult to express them in a way other people will understand. As Sudhanshu Grover, an autistic woman from India, says of her childhood and adulthood: "what I thought, I could not express in words."

This difficulty can be the result of many things going on in the person's mind. In some, it is dealing with physical surroundings that makes communication difficult. In others, it is self-consciousness. In someone like Deb Wrightson, an autistic woman from northeast England, it is a constant noise inside her head many autistic people can relate to. "I have a strong internal monologue, and my brain never seems to switch off," she said. "I'm always thinking about what I've read, saw, done, and making connections between things."

This difficulty with social communication can sometimes be mistaken as being anti-social. On the contrary, most autistic people crave human connection as much as anyone else; it's just that, as Wrightson shows, their brains are often just doing different things than what neurotypical ones do, which can make that connection harder.

Many autistic people spend a lot of time alone, and sometimes they are happy to do so. But the struggle with successfully connecting to other people can bring about lifelong issues with self-esteem because communication is the building block of human connection.[1] Strategies to connect with others are often either consciously learned through therapy and programs like social skills classes or gradually adopted through life experience. Noam Grossman, an autistic educator in Israel, relates to this through what he called his "main" communication issue, which is especially common among autistic people. "You're trying to find your words, and you want to create a whole sentence which needs to be comprehensible before [you] even say it," he said. "I'm second-guessing myself before I'm even talking. I'm not sure if people will understand me, so I'm not speaking before I'm speaking, which is very weird."

Someone could read this and think, "Well that's just being careful with what you say, what's different about that?" In the autistic context, however, this skill, which in its most pre-practiced forms is sometimes called "scripting" by the autistic community, is not applied for good manners alone. It is essential to staying in the basic good graces of other people.

If the natural answer to "How are you doing?" is a monologue that bores the other person, and an autistic person knows what they do is boring, they will then feel they have to stop, which requires a lot of conscious effort. This can be a real struggle.

What comes naturally to an autistic person can be wildly at odds with how a group of neurotypicals interact. If someone like Grossman or many other autistic people does not think enough in advance, the scale of the miscues could significantly lessen the quality of their relationships with other people, including potentially losing friends.

There are some significant ways this can happen, though this list is by no means exhaustive:

- **One-sided conversation**: The ways autistic people express their interests, which will be covered more in the "restricted and repetitive behaviours" chapter, can be off-putting. The clinical community can call this tendency "monologuing," while the autistic community can call it "infodumping."[2] Autistic people can talk for a long time about a subject of interest that is deeply exciting and stress relieving for them, but it can lead to blank stares and eventual annoyance by other people, especially if they are not interested in the topic.

However, this can also be true even if the other person *is* interested in the topic, but it is not talked about with conventional social rules in mind. Going to a symphony and talking about the piece with a newly met stranger by engaging in a ten-minute monologue about its complete history can lead to blank stares.

- **Reading the room**: Autistic children and adults are more likely to correct someone's mistakes, even sometimes harshly and in public. The first instinct for many autistic people is to deal with the truth. Despite what a neurotypical may feel, it is not usually the intention of an autistic person to embarrass anyone by doing this. They may only recognize what they did to someone's feelings after they have been told.[3] The same tendency can take place with regards to honesty in general. There was an incident when Donald Triplett, Kanner's first patient, told a pep rally at his community college that their team was going to lose a football game, much to the displeasure of a booing crowd.[4] But Triplett was just telling it as he saw it; it didn't occur to him to worry about how the crowd thought.
- **Misunderstanding intentions**: They can mistake a person's intentions or the mood of a group. It is common to lack at least an instinctive understanding of sarcasm. It is also common for autistic people to not understand the meaning of non-literal speech, such as implication, idiom, or metaphor, though some recent research noted this can be more variable among autistic people.[5] It is also common for them to not catch someone's tone of voice or adapt their speech to reflect the demographics of others, the formality, or the context of the occasion.[6]

Mistakes like this may result in awkwardness or polite correction. Sometimes, if a neurotypical person does not understand how autistic people think, or the mistake results in deep hurt, it can be much more consequential, like the end of a connection with someone. Some of these kinds of missteps, like not picking up on the fact a person is bored and doesn't want to talk to them, can lead to an autistic person believing a relationship is closer than it is.[7] This is particularly true if the other person's feelings are not made clear, like if the person nevertheless entertains the conversation and doesn't say they want to stop talking.

- **Respecting physical space**: They can intrude into a person's personal space in a way that is off-putting or even intimidating.

This could be physically getting too close to someone or messaging them too often on social media without enough of a prior relationship.[8] Conversely, they can also be withdrawn and disengaged from a group of people in a way that can make them seem anti-social.[9]

- **Non-spoken cues**: Autistic people's non-spoken communication and tendencies can be viewed as peculiar and off-putting to some neurotypical people who do not understand autism. Lack of eye contact, while not itself a sign of autism, was noticed in autistic people from the earliest clinical research. Hans Asperger said of one of his students that "his eye gaze was strikingly odd."[10] Other traits can include toe walking, a stiff gait, an apparent lack of facial expression, and a monotone voice.

These traits can be extremely off-putting for neurotypical people, who may feel that an autistic person is self-centred, odd, naïve, and unfeeling towards others. Those who think this way do not understand that these tendencies reflect a lot of innate thought patterns. How autistic people communicate makes sense when those patterns are understood. These have to do with how to cope with thinking more literally than neurotypicals do, or seeing patterns in places most people do not, or seeing the world in terms of references to their interests, or understanding how people see change. These can all come out in speech, and it makes sense if people care to dig deeper.

Just as there are selfish neurotypicals, there are selfish autistic people, but as a group, they are unlikely to be more selfish than anyone else, at least if selfish is defined as serving one's own needs while being indifferent or hostile to other people. Their mistakes are not inherently reflections of selfishness or malice. They are more likely preoccupied with intellectually dealing with parts of conversation that are natural to neurotypicals. They are not as focused on the other person because they are more worried about managing what they are doing, just as a beginner driver sometimes focuses on the mechanics of operating the car before they intuitively attend to what is happening on the road.

These skills can get better with practice, and evidence shows that most autistic people manage these skills better as adults.[11] However, practiced effort is always clumsier and more prone to error than innate ability. Social communication in humans is highly complex, context-dependent, and often counterintuitive to an autistic brain, so even the most neurotypical-seeming autistic adults still struggle to adapt.

The process of learning how to avoid these mistakes is not just intellectually difficult but also painful. Autistic people often understand they are different from the time they are little kids, and it can take years of embarrassment and hurt to learn even some of the rules necessary to avoid making mistakes once they become adults. At this stage, such experiences can even be traumatic.[12]

## Adolescence and Adult Difficulties

Social communication issues have similar origins but often take different forms in childhood and adulthood. As with all humans, puberty is the start of many characteristics of autistic people that last for the rest of their lives. One of these is self-consciousness. Just as neurotypical adolescents are gaining more self-consciousness, autistic adolescents are too. The difference is that autistic adolescents can start to be more self-conscious about their autistic traits, seeing that they can be off-putting to others. This can be particularly true in autistic people with higher IQs, showing that "high functioning" can sometimes be a curse as well as a blessing.[13] This can lead to feelings of depression and intense self-consciousness.[14]

"Below the age of twelve, I was never lonely even though I didn't have friends," said M.,[15] a middle-aged autistic woman living in Canada. "I was always very occupied with something or other in the environment. I was always outside; I was always on my bicycle, or I was climbing trees or doing some kind of experiment or fixing something. So it didn't bother me whether people wanted to talk to me or not. But when I got to be a teenager, then it, of course, it started to bug me."

Sometimes autism is even diagnosed in adolescence or adulthood based on these issues. This has been particularly noticed in clinical settings with teenage girls and women.[16] At this time, social requirements become more complex, and the autistic person's challenges are more easily exposed. This sudden difficulty can be jarring, but it can also lead to a breakthrough in identifying a potential autism diagnosis.[17]

For children, social interaction is usually limited to their family, teachers, and friends. Their interactions with adults are usually in more predictable, controlled environments, like regular dinners and asking for chores to be done. Social skills at this age are largely limited to shared interests and game playing.[18] This time is formative, but relatively simple socially.

Later in life, social interaction becomes more complicated. There are romantic relationships, which lead to larger in-law family connections, as well as workplace interactions, caretaker-type exchanges with parents, relationships with their own children, and even contacts with strangers, whom children are often discouraged from talking to.

This is all on top of conventional friendships. Even friendships can become more complicated as people become adults. The changing circumstances of work and location mean maintaining friendships as an adult is more difficult. People get married and have children of their own, meaning less time for friends, and commitments to jobs and important family matters make their lives even busier.

Autistic people, regardless of age, tend to find change unusually disorienting and distressing. While ending friendships is sad for anyone, autistic people are more likely to have especially intense feelings towards people they have become close to. They can feel it unusually strongly when the nature of a relationship changes.[19]

This can be explained partially through temperament and partially through experience.

By temperament, apart from change, autistic children can tend towards clinginess with friends. If a friend is playing with another friend, they can take it as a sign of personal rejection.[20] This is not due to a creepy or abusive tendency, as some neurotypicals might interpret. It can be out of desperation, a feeling of a sense of betrayal, or just simply how they see friendship.

A neurotypical may see two friends as just two different people that they play with sometimes individually, but an autistic person may see a friend as one person having a kind of special bond with another. It is not quite seen as a romantic relationship, but as an analogy, there are some similarities.[21] This tendency can also lead to an autistic person misunderstanding the other person's point of view about the nature and strength of a relationship. They may see a friendship where the neurotypical person sees the two as acquaintances — at most.[22]

By the time these autistic children are adults, many if not most can learn to understand what is going on and control this impulse to a socially acceptable level. Even with these skills, however, an innate tendency towards a certain kind of loyalty can remain.[23]

Because of this difference in neurology and expectation, an autistic person can be confused by a friend who is talking with them less than before or not at all. They can wonder if they have done something wrong, or — even worse — if *they* are fundamentally wrong. This can increase anxiety and depression, and there can be an intense need for closure and clarity.[24] This tendency is not true of all autistic people, of course, but it can help explain certain kinds of behaviour in friendships that a neurotypical person may misunderstand.

*It can be crucial to be direct about where someone stands with an autistic person because of this difference.* If an autistic person is not told that a friendship is over, they may not pick up the signs that it is. Neurotypicals can often "feel" the changes during a friendship. While it may be sad, they are more likely to adapt because of their innate understanding of how these situations work, and they can move on more easily.

An explanation that change is coming, as well as why, goes a long way towards keeping an autistic person secure. It may take some patience and explaining on the part of a friend to make understandable what is going on, but clear goals and commitments that are followed up on often help an autistic person in dealing with these issues.

An autistic person's experience is also critical. Almost all people gain at least some of their sense of self-worth by how people perceive them. For autistic adults, there can be a history of failed or strained friendships and relationships because their traits have led to people rejecting them. For particularly unlucky autistic people, this can also include their family.

Some of this behaviour can also be linked to fear of abandonment. They have experienced rejection so often that they are desperate not to have it repeated. Counterintuitively for that autistic person, these kinds of clingy behaviours can lead to even more rejection. The kinds of social experiences and development most neurotypicals take for granted may have either been insufficient or completely denied to autistic people.

Trauma can also play a major role in how autistic people approach relationships. Because of their innate brain structure and lack of social experiences, they can be more naïve than a person of a similar chronological age.

Due to this, autistic women are more likely to get into abusive relationships because they will not recognize the signs of an abusive man that a neurotypical woman would. Men can also fall prey to being victim to other people; in childhood, this could be bullies, and in adulthood, this could be "friends" or family who want to take advantage of them. Transgender people, whether neurotypical or autistic, face disproportionate levels of trauma from society in general.

This trauma can also contribute to mistrust and withdrawal. Autistic people can try to cope with this in several ways. British clinical psychologist Tony Attwood lists depression (which can include withdrawal from others), escape into imagination, denial of even being autistic, arrogance (often regarding intellectual ability), and trying to imitate their peers to cover up their autistic traits as potential coping mechanisms for handling social rejection.[25] These are not necessarily universal traits among autistic adults; many never feel a need to resort to these coping mechanisms. While this list is a good start, it also leads to more questions than it answers, including: Why does a person resort to these mechanisms? How does a person who has been rejected repeatedly gain self-worth? Also, how do they gain self-worth when the reasons they are rejected are for traits largely outside of their control?

People with diminished self-worth are more likely to have bad outcomes, with suicide being among the worst. People need a sense of self-worth not just to thrive but to live. If someone is rejected by others, they can find purpose in something else. For intellectually minded autistic people, this can be a certain conceit in their own intelligence and commitment to their interests. For others, it can mean an outright denial of their autism and desire to fit in at all costs.

One of these coping mechanisms is even more sympathetic. Tony Attwood has publicly told a story of a seven-year-old girl who talked out loud to a girl named Sarah, who did not exist. She was referred to him by school staff who thought she had schizophrenia, showing how history repeats itself, with people making the same mistakes again and again. When Attwood questioned the girl about her "hallucination," she said they talked about the school rules and the principal, in other words, the kinds of subjects any girl her age would discuss. Attwood then realized this was not a hallucinating person with schizophrenia but a lonely autistic girl. Sarah was an imaginary friend, created to cope with the fact she had no friends at school. Autistic adults do not usually have imaginary friends, but a vivid imagination and preoccupation with fantasy can still exist, which if properly honed, can help them lead a creative life.[26]

Adolescents and adults who become extremely interested in fiction may have done so because they were feeling a loneliness like the seven-year-old girl's. However, anyone who has met autistic people with these interests also knows that this is a powerful way they can bond with other people. This is how a coping mechanism for dealing with rejection can become a healthy way of bonding with others. This is true of many autistic people's passions.

However, in regular scenarios with people who are not selected for interest, like a workplace, it can be challenging and exhausting to maintain connections with others.

Examples of all these coping mechanisms will be covered throughout this book. The earliest motivations for using the mechanisms at all have roots in aspects of autistic communication, and the disconnect with neurotypicals, that well predates the experiences autistic people have as adults.

## Empathy, Theory of Mind, and the Sally–Anne Test/Double Empathy Problem

Of all the ways to show the cultural side of autism, there may be none better than to look at the Sally–Anne test and the double empathy problem. Simon Baron-Cohen, a young Cambridge University researcher working under more seasoned researchers Uta Frith and Alan Leslie in the 1980s, developed a test that is widely used to help diagnose autistic children. The Sally–Anne test, as it became known, consists of two dolls named Sally and Anne, a box, a basket, and a marble. It starts when Sally puts the marble in a basket and walks away. While she is gone, Anne takes the marble and puts it in the box. The participant is then asked a critical question: Where does Sally *think* the marble is. Of course, the right answer is the basket. But how do people know that?

Findings that pre-dated Baron-Cohen's test, especially from Heinz Wimmer and Jozef Perner's experiments in 1983 with how children relate to puppets, which were credited with pioneering this kind of test, showed that most children over age four could understand and get the right answer to a question like this.[27] The tests that Baron-Cohen, Frith, and Leslie conducted between 1985, where Sally and Anne were represented by dolls and the scenario was role-played, and 1988, where actors played out the scenario, however, showed one exception.[28]

Autistic children were found to have failed the Sally–Anne test more often than non-autistic children. Children with Down syndrome, who often have an intellectual disability, and neurotypical children mostly got the answer right, but not the autistic children.

The non-autistic kids, averaging around age seven in Baron-Cohen's study, were also older than most of the non-autistic children, aged three or four, which is when the ability to understand other people's intentions usually starts to develop in neurotypical people.[29]

What this test showed was that failing the Sally–Anne test was not due to general intellectual disability. If true, the Down syndrome participants would have been more likely to fail.

Social understanding is different from intellect. The ability to understand another person's thoughts and intentions is different from whether someone could read quickly or solve math problems.

Theory of mind is often confused with empathy, but empathy is about seeing how someone is feeling and being able to relate to, and share in, those feelings. Seeing someone who is writhing in pain and coming to their aid is an action that indicates empathy.[30] Autistic people do not usually have issues with empathy — quite the contrary. It is more often reported that they can feel what others feel *too much*, to the point where it can provoke crippling anxiety and perseveration (the continual involuntary repetition of a thought or behaviour).

Instead, theory of mind is the ability to imagine what another person is *thinking*, not feeling. To avoid confusion, psychologists sometimes use the terms "affective empathy," which autistic people do not usually lack, and "cognitive empathy," which autistic people more frequently do lack. By contrast, a clinical psychopath is a person with the reverse problem. They understand other people, they just don't care about them. They use their understanding of people to manipulate them.[31]

Theory of mind abilities in adults are tested more through everyday circumstance. Autistic adults can usually pass the Sally–Anne test when looking at it and thinking it through, but they can still have false beliefs in real-life scenarios, which are rooted in not being able to understand what another person might be thinking.[32]

*Therefore, an explanation of what is going on can help make reality clearer to an autistic person.* They *might* then understand what they need to do.

Some people object to theory of mind as a valid concept in social science, but the problem for them is that the evidence for theory of mind is now substantial. A large meta-analysis of 830 studies conducted from

1983 to 2019 showed not just that theory of mind exists, but that it can be broken down into seven main areas with thirty-nine subcategories.[33]

Psychologists now know a lot about theory of mind. There are questions about the use of false belief tests like the Sally–Anne test to establish theory of mind, such as from Paul Bloom at Yale University.[34] But the idea of a theory of mind separate from IQ, and indeed from empathy, is now well-established, and it is by conventional definitions lacking in many autistic people.

However, another way of looking at theory of mind has also received notoriety, especially among the autistic community. In 2012, autistic sociology professor Damian Milton, then at the University of Birmingham, published a paper proposing an idea called the "double empathy problem."[35] He proposed that autistic people understand other autistic people better than they understand neurotypicals, while neurotypicals understand each other more than they understand autistic people. The mismatch of brain wiring causes a misunderstanding when two people from these different groups meet. This mismatch is the core emphasis for Milton, whereas the Sally–Anne test focuses on an autistic person's inability to see what is in another's head. Milton calls this disconnect a "mismatch of salience," which was also the title of one of his books, because it reflects a difference in what autistic and neurotypical people automatically view as important in social interaction and even in the world.

In short, according to Milton, it is better to think of autistic and neurotypical people as two different cultures who share the same planet and must understand each other, rather than a sick group that must conform to a healthy one. He developed this theory, based on his work in the 1990s, specifically to counteract theories like Baron-Cohen's.

"I was reading the Theory of Mind, Simon Baron-Cohen type work . . . I saw the Theory of Mind stuff as partial at best," said Milton. "It's a very one-way view at seeing the interaction . . . very othering of the autistic way of being." He says neurotypical social conventions, such as maintaining eye contact and reading between the lines, which autistic people are more likely to struggle with, are factors that unfairly exclude them from social life. To Milton, it is as important for neurotypical people to understand autistic social cues as it is for autistic people to understand neurotypical ones.

It is crucial to understand the double empathy problem in its original writing as something related to activism and philosophy more than science.

Milton has a deep social justice component in his academic work, and this idea should be considered as part of that analysis.

For instance, in his 2012 paper, Milton says that academics who want to integrate autistic people into society are "informed by research that champions the use of the randomised controlled trial, yet discounts the subjective experiences of those who identify as being on the autism spectrum themselves as worthy of rigorous academic study."[36] This does not make the double empathy problem wrong, but its origins should be noted, as it was never intended to be science and should not be taken as such.

Milton said this phrasing was "a bit harsh" and favours interdisciplinary work on autism, including with scientists. To be clear, Milton is not anti-science. His overall point, however, about looking at lived experiences of autistic people, is clearly a major focus of not only his work but also many disability studies and other social science analyses of autism-related issues.

There is some tension with mainstream science on this point, as lived experience and particularly anecdotal evidence are often viewed with skepticism in a scientific context because they lack reliability and validity, and rely on the subjectivity of the person's account.

Whatever someone may think of the origins of his ideas, some experiments have concluded that Milton's theory may have validity in more scientific types of analysis. Work by academics like Rosanna Eddy, Elizabeth Shepard, Brett Heasman, and Noah Sasson have shown that neurotypical people also had a difficult time reading the intentions of autistic people.[37] Heasman and Alex Gillespie have written about miscommunication between autistic people and neurotypical family members.[38] Sasson's work has also found that neurotypicals are likely to make false snap judgments of autistic people's behaviour that do not fit into what the autistic person believes they are doing themselves. Luca Casartelli's research shows neurotypical people often mistake the intentions of autistic children by misunderstanding their motor movements.[39] These results support the earlier idea that autistic people are more likely to be falsely seen as liars by neurotypicals based on their social presentation.

The evidence for the other part of Milton's thesis, that autistic people better understand each other, is somewhat limited. However, an article in the prestigious academic journal *Autism*, based on interviews with only twelve autistic participants, showed there has been some subjectivity-based research to suggest that they feel more comfortable around other autistic people.[40]

There is still a lot more research left to do on this question. Its overall effect has profound implications by directly addressing how autistic people function in the world. Accepting the work of Baron-Cohen but not Milton has been seen to imply that autistic people must conform to a neurotypical way of socializing. Many self-advocates believe this interpretation and regard it as a justification for trying to "change" autistic people. Accepting the conclusions of Milton and not Baron-Cohen means it is most important for neurotypicals to understand autistic people. Self-advocates believe this is particularly true given the pain and misunderstanding autistic people can experience. It is also seen as a more useful way to understand people, though some critics will say that it is not a view of science and therefore may have limited validity.

There is another alternative, which is that this may not be an either-or problem. It is possible that autistic people can have difficulties understanding most people while acknowledging that they have something in common with a smaller group of people like them, and that neurotypicals do not understand this group. The overall body of knowledge may lead to suggest that there must be some give and take on both sides. Autistic people should try to understand the way most people think and behave accordingly, at least to the best of their ability. But society should also understand how to identify autistic people, keep in mind the difficulties they face, and try to interact with them in a friendly and non-stigmatizing way.

The potential lack of conflict between these two ideas may also be reflected in Baron-Cohen himself, as he has come out on the side of some neurodiversity-minded ideas on numerous occasions, even if theory of mind is not seen by some self-advocates as a neurodiversity-minded idea. He suggested that autism spectrum disorder should be renamed autism spectrum *condition* rather than disorder, as it is in the DSM, which he considers to be a less stigmatizing term. He believes this does more to reflect autistic people's strengths as well as challenges.[41] He has also written in support of a mixed view of a social and medical model of disability.[42]

Baron-Cohen published a book in 2020, *The Pattern Seekers: How Autism Drives Human Invention*, that celebrates autistic traits in human invention going back to primitive history. This parrots Temple Grandin's old saying, of course said provocatively and not literally, that if there were no autistic people, human beings would still be in caves around campfires socializing.[43] The book notes the struggles of autistic people as well, but strongly reflects their strengths.

This is a point where Baron-Cohen and Milton are likely to agree. In some circles, their views are presented as something to accept fully in one way or the other, but the gifts of autistic people are evident in both of their writings when taken overall, even if the language, approach, and methods may differ.

This issue in some ways sums up all the other issues of social communication that matter to autistic people covered earlier. The ability to empathize is often considered a core human trait. The lack of ability to empathize is often considered one of the traits most off-putting to others, so it matters that autistic people are not falsely stereotyped in this way. The lack of understanding autistic people can sometimes have about what others think and intend, and the lack of neurotypical people's ability to understand what an autistic person thinks and understands causes fundamental barriers to communication.

Mutual understanding can help improve communication. Gaining this for a neurotypical can come with reading but will be powerful with enough exposure to autistic people. Understanding and getting to know them may take some patience at first, but while they may initially struggle to relate, enough exposure can reveal a person who is a valuable friend. If this is a double empathy problem, autistic people can also learn a lot from the perspectives of neurotypicals, though what they will learn will likely be different. This will take more than just curiosity. For many autistic people, given their negative experiences socializing, this can even be an act of courage and faith. There will be troubles and judgment, but most people are not out to harm autistic people, and doing something challenging and rewarding is one of the great long-lasting joys of life.

Regardless of which perspective one takes, knowing more people and really trying to understand them is deeply important. If mutual understanding is a core problem at the heart of neurotypical/autistic interaction, bridging this issue may at least get people on the right track.

## A Few Brief Tips on How to Bridge This Gap

If there is indeed a fundamental "mismatch of salience" or "theory of mind" problem, then the question is how to engage in a conversation with an autistic person if you're a neurotypical. There are some starting points.

*The first is to begin any conversation with an autistic person understanding that their differences mean communication will likely be a slower process.* If the person communicates through means other than spoken word, such as a speech-to-word machine, this will be especially obvious. Even for autistic people who are fluent verbally, the differences in understanding will mean that some things that a neurotypical takes for granted may have to be explained. They may have to be more conscious about using non-literal phrases, if this is something an autistic person struggles with. Sometimes these phrases can slip out, and a quick explanation is usually sufficient for an autistic person to understand and to carry on the conversation.

Likewise, if an autistic person makes an idiosyncratic reference that a neurotypical person doesn't understand, such as a reference to a favourite television show or comic, it is not offensive to calmly ask what they are talking about. They are using something that is within their own frame of reference, just as all humans do. Like being in a different culture, the references may sometimes not compute.

Given the degree of passion an autistic person can have for their subject, taking an interest in the subject enough to at least ask questions can make an autistic person extremely excited.

Displays of communication outside of conversation may also be expressed differently. An autistic person may not immediately understand social customs intuitively. If a neurotypical person wants an autistic person to help them with dishwashing or cleaning the floor, gently asking will usually work. It should also be understood that this may be something that needs to be repeated every time they want help, not something that is set as a general expectation.

Neurotypical people should also understand that autistic people's threshold for communication, especially in a traditional neurotypical sense, might be lower. They are not being rude by shutting down or excusing themselves; it's just part of who they are. Part of how it feels to be autistic is trying to comprehend the world around them, which they can do to varying degrees of success. A little bit of understanding of how an autistic person is will go a long way.

They may find being in a loud restaurant too overwhelming for long periods of time, they may find the cognitive work of lengthy conversation too overwhelming, or they might not like or understand more sophisticated forms of communication, like non-literal or non-spoken speech, especially jokes. This is where one potential area for shared experience, as well as pain, can lie.

## Humour

In the early days of autism research, there was some question as to whether a group of generally literal thinking, non-socially skilled people could appreciate something as non-literal and socially bonding as humour. For a long time, the answer was thought to be no.

This belief was even held and perpetuated by Hans Asperger, who said his children were "rarely relaxed and carefree and never achieve that particular wisdom and deep intuitive human understanding that underlie genuine humor."[44] Despite being ahead of his time on many other topics related to autism, he badly misunderstood his children here, in part, due to his metrics. Asperger once tried testing his children's sense of humour by showing them funny cartoons, and when they did not find them funny, this deficit was what Asperger concluded. This probably says more about Asperger, or the cartoons, than it did about autistic people.

It is now recognized that autistic people can have well-developed senses of humour. Some even get to the level of professional comedians, such as Canadian Michael McCreary, who bases most of his comedy on his own autism. His humour is self-deprecating, uplifting, and full of observation, as demonstrated in one of his signature bits.

> I even got my own joke superhero out of it. His name was Socially Awkward Man. [Said in a dramatic "faster than a speeding bullet" voice] Clad in a speedo and a balaclava. Nothing bothers Socially Awkward Man. With the incomparable ability to withstand changing the subject, oblivious to personal space, more tenacious than a telemarketer, able to create embarrassing pauses

> with a single proclamation — hey! [points ahead of him] I can see Uranus [your anus] from here.[45]

It is also not just McCreary who does this. Among others, Bethany Black,[46] Dan Ackroyd,[47] and Hannah Gadsby[48] have also been diagnosed autistic. Even Jerry Seinfeld, one of the most popular comedians in American history, has said publicly he believes he is on the spectrum.[49]

What can be different is that the style of humour can be unlike that of most neurotypical people, sometimes depending more on wordplay or humour involving punch lines, in contrast to what is expected, as is even seen in the McCreary bit.

More common kinds of conversational or non-literal humour, like irony and sarcasm, might be more challenging to understand for autistic people.[50] Just as they may understand a non-funny, non-literal phrase like "call me at any time," as "call me even at 3:30 in the morning," they may take a sarcastic question like "Isn't that nice?" to be genuine inquiry. This is by no means universal. Sometimes, the issue is understanding humorous intent in another person, not failing to understand the concept of humour and even being able to use it themselves.

"Sometimes, unless it's obvious, I do fail to read sarcasm," said Charlie Sansom, a young Canadian autistic university student. "Which is ironic because I am a fairly sarcastic guy." What Sansom is saying is probably quite relatable to many autistic people. It is not as if the idea of irony or sarcasm is beyond their comprehension; many autistic people can use it, never mind understand it. It is just that they may struggle to grasp it *in real time.*

What often varies between autistic and neurotypical people is how fast they process certain kinds of humour. The joke can occur more slowly in an autistic person's mind.[51] A common autistic experience is that they may say something funny or interesting, but they may say it well after the time when it might have struck the right chord with the group. The timing may be off because they will not process the conversation as quickly as their peers. This does not mean the wit is absent entirely. Autistic people can make jokes and do laugh at what they find funny, even if their humour is idiosyncratic.

However, there can also be other differences. The level of maturity of the humour can sometimes be contrary to expectations. Since autism is a developmental condition, what thirteen-year-old autistic people find funny may be more commonly found funny in younger neurotypical children, like saying "poop" or "pee" in a comical way. This can also be true of what thirteen-year-old autistic people understand in terms of profanity or sexuality, which are often growing sources of humour in adolescence and adulthood.[52]

This naïveté can sometimes be taken advantage of, for example, jokes like asking a male autistic adolescent "Do you like schlong?" which is slang for penis. When asked to define "schlong," they may say "schlong is chocolate cake," to which they then may respond, "Sure, I like schlong," which then results in intense laughter at the autistic adolescent's expense.

This kind of teasing then shows how missing certain aspects of humour can go from awkwardness to bullying, and then why this subject can be no laughing matter. Although a moment like this can just be intended as playful teasing, it can also be bullying and taking advantage of someone's vulnerability. It is crucial to find that line, especially with autistic people who may be more vulnerable. Crossing it too often can lead to lasting psychological damage.[53]

How each autistic individual copes with these issues varies depending on their own personality and level of understanding. *Autistic adults should not be treated as if they are innocent and vulnerable children, especially when they clearly are not.* Autistic people can be more vulnerable to certain kinds of missteps regarding humour because they may not immediately understand what is happening.

Certain jokes that are obvious to most will not be obvious to autistic people, and may be received literally, not at all, or in a way that a neurotypical does not expect. *Giving calm clarifications can be extremely helpful for autistic people, especially if they obviously don't get the joke.*

These misunderstandings in social communication in adulthood extend well beyond just not getting jokes. What about in areas where the stakes are much higher?

## Medical Misunderstandings

Communication errors are even more likely to happen in specialized and stressful settings, such as dealing with the health-care system. Many autistic people have difficulties expressing themselves, including stating their needs and feelings, which is essential to advocating for one's own health, and this can make health-care access more difficult for them than for neurotypicals. This is even more important because autistic people are more likely to have regular experience with the health-care system because of the increased risk of mental and physical health issues.[54]

A lot of autistic people tell negative stories about the medical system. Their experience getting a diagnosis can include long wait times, the high cost, and especially potential misunderstandings. Some autistic people are misdiagnosed because of these issues, while others who should be diagnosed are missed by everyone including themselves.[55]

One study from Europe in 2020 tested a random sample of 161 adults who evaluators identified as being autistic. On average, it took eleven years from the first psychiatric session to diagnosis as an adult. About two-thirds were initially given a diagnosis other than autism, indicating the difficulty with diagnosis for adults even today.[56]

These problems happen because of failures of communication and misunderstanding. This is also more likely to happen in adults because psychiatric professionals are still more familiar with autism in children, if they are familiar with autism at all.[57] By adulthood, there is an increased likelihood that autism-related traits are mistaken for personality disorders, mood disorders, and other conditions that usually show themselves in adulthood.[58] It is more straightforward to diagnose a child as being autistic, which is one reason why early intervention is ideal.

*This should not dissuade adults who believe they are autistic from getting a diagnosis.* Receiving an accurate autism diagnosis at any time in life is life-changing. It is just that missed diagnoses and the communication challenges that help cause them are more likely in adulthood, so communication from both parties must be particularly clear and asking a lot of questions becomes even more paramount.

Apart from events that happen once or twice in a lifetime, like diagnosis, there are issues with communication in the day-to-day encounters with medical professionals. These communication issues also mean that more patience and time may be necessary when problems do happen, and the recommendation is that an autistic person and their medical care providers establish a strong relationship.[59] If someone knows an autistic person well, they may be able to understand them better.

Issues with autistic people accessing the health-care system have long been well-known. A 2005 report from Ontario recommended a litany of changes that would make it easier for them to access the health-care system. The ones that were communication-oriented included enhancement of professional expertise, which has just been covered, and an increased use of teleconferencing. This can be helpful because autistic people may be more comfortable talking to a doctor at home than in a hospital due to the inherent sensory issues and stress associated with health-care settings.[60]

Many other recommendations from this report and other sources will be covered in part 2. However, these two recommendations speak to Milton's idea that understanding autistic people is a two-way street. Making the world easier for them to communicate in will improve how they experience the world, even in stressful situations such as handling their medical issues.

Dealing with the health-care system is particularly relevant to older autistic adults, defined as those over forty and especially those over sixty, because they are most likely to use the medical system. Their experiences, however, indicate there can be additional communication problems that can make accessing health care more difficult.

This group is chronically understudied in research in general. Wenn Lawson, an autistic expert on the condition at Birmingham University, wrote a book specifically about older autistic adults in 2015. He sums it up this way:

> Older individuals with ASC [author's note: ASC stands for autism spectrum condition, a way of naming autism spectrum disorder seen as more respectful of autistic people] may not know about or understand those expectations. When is it the right time to talk? Do I tell the receptionist my problems? How long do I wait if my appointment is for a certain time, but that time has come and gone? What if I need treatment from another doctor or a specialist? If I get told "You are seeing the doctor," but they send me to a different doctor, what does this mean? Are they both "the doctor?" Will the doctor speak to me in terms I understand, or will they treat me like I'm stupid?
>
> Older people with ASC depend on professionals to be informed and to know how to share the information

> with them. The individual needs to give the general practitioner time to get to know them, so should aim to visit the same GP each time.[61]

This kind of familiarity can be critical because each autistic person has a unique way of communicating. A constant, familiar relationship allows an autistic person to be more comfortable with someone they know as well as a medical practitioner to better understand the person and how to talk to and treat them.

Lawson believes that older autistic people admitted to hospital should get a single room or, at bare minimum, a room with a curtain around it to reduce noise stimulation. Particular care should be taken to explain every step before anything is done for them, to reduce the likelihood of confusion and disorientation.[62]

This can be true of autistic people in general, not just older ones. If time and space is available, dealing with an autistic person's care more slowly and methodically can make a world of difference. But with older people who may have a complicated set of needs and who may become disoriented, this is crucial. All of this is even more applicable to autistic people who do not speak at all or have profound communication challenges, when even more extra patience will be necessary.

In many cases, more obviously autistic people will likely attend medical appointments accompanied by a caregiver, who could be a parent, a sibling, or a personal support worker. This person will likely know better how the autistic person communicates and can interpret their individual ways of communicating that health-care staff might not be familiar with.

This is true not just in health care but also in their entire lives. A major challenge in day-to-day life for autistic people with significant speech difficulties is making themselves understood through non-speaking means. If people are not easily understood, they can be easily dismissed. This is still a critical issue for this group. Thankfully, there are tools to help.

## Augmented and Assisted Communication

For many autistic people, communication challenges can be so profound, whether all the time or only in some situations, that they may have to use forms of technology to assist them and even to help them develop language. This technology is called augmented and assisted communication, often shortened to AAC. This issue has become salient enough that access to AAC has even become one of the fifteen pillars of the Communication Bill of Rights, which the National Joint Committee for the Communication Needs of Persons with Severe Disabilities created.[63]

AAC use is best known in cases of autism where the person is non-speaking or minimally speaking. For these people, communication issues are not just a matter of failing to bond or avoiding social embarrassment. It affects every aspect of daily life. These inabilities can be extremely frustrating, which is linked to higher-than-expected rates of depression even in more obviously presenting autistic children.[64] In autistic people in general, rates of depression are high by adulthood, but in this group, it can present even earlier.

The best way to think about non-speaking autistic people can be to consider them as someone whose general language is underdeveloped. If a twelve-month-old child had a medical problem, it would not be wise to depend on them to verbally describe their pain in order to determine how to treat them. The best way would be to figure out *their* system.

There are other cues the person could be giving that "say" what needs to be "said." Families of non-speaking or minimally speaking autistic people will realize over time what they mean by certain echoed phrases, gestures, or emotional reactions. However, non-speaking or minimally speaking autistic people can communicate in some ways that are a little easier for those who do not know them. This is often where AAC comes in.

These devices are often categorized as low-tech, medium-tech, and high-tech. Low-tech usually means non-electronic forms of communication. These can include cardboard picture boards that have an array of pictures with accompanying words that the person points to indicating what they need. Medium-tech can be an electronic board that uses simple speech commands, like pressing a button that says "I want *x*." High-tech AAC can include electronic devices that create more complex speech. Some non-speaking autistic people can even type out their thoughts with high-tech word processors, including speech-to-word software.

The same person can also use a mix of different kinds of communication tools, depending on the circumstances. These kinds of tools have proved to be highly effective for children and young adults and give non-speaking autistic adults more ability to communicate needs.[65] But it is not a substitute for speech.

One of the things that meta-analyses of AAC reveal is that, beyond commands like "I want a cookie" or "I'm feeling tired," the ability for nonspeaking autistic people to have "socially valid" speech, which allows more typical interactions with others, is less well-established. Nevertheless, the usefulness of AAC is even more profound than many professionals believed even a generation ago. AAC was once thought to be a last resort for autistic people who could not communicate in some other way. It was believed that dependency on these devices would slow their growth in communication.

Quite to the contrary, as the evidence suggests now.[66] AAC can help even *increase* the rate that people pick up and develop speech, though this also depends on the person using it. AAC is also used by autistic people who have more speech initially but use a device for specific situations. This technology can be a method of last resort if they are in a situation where they are getting emotional to the point of a shutdown or meltdown, which can be a matter of life and death.

Some adult autistic people carry a card indicating their diagnosis if they are confronted by the police, as there are studies that show about one-third of them are likely to have an encounter with the police.[67] Autistic people are more likely to be stopped and have awkward encounters with police than neurotypicals, and these interactions are stressful experiences for people more likely to have issues regulating their emotions or getting the right words out.[68] Lack of typical communication and visible signs of stress can send an unsettling signal to a police officer, especially if they have no idea who the person is and why they are less than ideally responsive. Having the card is meant to calm these situations. It is a less cognitively intensive way of saying what is going on to a police officer, and the officer can then deal with the situation accordingly.

Other kinds of signs are also used to indicate how willing and able a person is to interact in specialized settings like autism conferences. People wearing a green sign means anyone can come up to talk to them, yellow means they will talk to people they know, and red means don't approach them to talk at all.[69] These signs are helpful because some autistic people have selective mutism, meaning they will speak to only some people and not others, often if the person is well-known to them. Selective mutism is not unique to autism, with limited data suggesting that only 8% of people with selective mutism are autistic, but it is more common among autistic people than in the general population.[70]

In specialized settings, where these rules are understood, such badges are affirming and helpful. For autistic people, it is a clear way to express their preferences and needs. For people unfamiliar with autism, it can also clearly show the variety of autistic culture. In ordinary life, however, this system is not used and understood. This is where other forms of AAC, like those others already listed, can help with navigating the world.

*These kinds of tools should be used as much as an autistic person feels they need it, and a neurotypical person can help by being patient and helping them master the use of an AAC.* Some AACs are relatively inexpensive, and as will be covered later, help is available for more expensive ones.

There are also areas of autistic life where no kind of AAC will ever be sufficient.

## Communication in Sex and Relationships

Managing communication issues in sex and relationships is difficult for everyone, but especially for autistic adults. The fundamental issues are largely the same, but the social and emotional tools that they have can be different. There may be more patience and understanding needed from both an autistic and neurotypical person.

One fundamental issue is that autistic adults can sometimes misunderstand signs of romantic interest because they lack experience or understanding. They may mistake general friendliness for romantic interest, and assume their own feelings and intentions are reciprocated.[71]

Autistic people can have other issues with how to engage in dating and sex. They may misunderstand boundaries and even take quality advice in a way that is not intended by the presenter. For example, asking for consent has been interpreted by some autistic men as going up to women they do not know and asking to touch their private parts.[72] This can seem perverted to an outsider, but inside the man's head, they are literally following a rule given by a sex education lesson. "If you want to engage in sexual activity with someone, ask for consent" is how the advice is often stated.

Given these assumptions, how this autistic person behaves can make sense. That autistic man may even believe that asking women this way can be responsible. However, he did not understand the unspoken and underlying assumption behind this sentence.

This is the way to break it down when talking to an autistic person: *think about what this bit of advice does not say, and then think about the literal-mindedness that autistic people can have and how this advice might be received.* Most neurotypical teenagers and young men would understand that this means asking someone after sexual interest has been established. These people are more likely to have the experience and innate understanding necessary to know this. Autistic people may misinterpret this and take it to mean asking anyone *they* want to have sex with, in the moment or otherwise.

This also applies to many other scenarios, especially involving boundaries. Misunderstandings for the autistic person can happen when they are casually approached by the person they are interested in sexually, leading to misunderstandings about when it is appropriate to contact them or be around them at all. Autistic people have sometimes not understood these boundaries, and people interacting with them have even believed them to be stalkers.

As stated earlier, sexual relationships are unusually complicated, especially for someone who has differences in social understanding. *In this situation, among others, it is often good to be as thorough and concrete with autistic people as possible because how they interpret advice may not be what the person giving it intends.* Explain what it means as literally as possible. It can also be a good idea to then ask them to repeat it, and then ask if there is any confusion.

This can be a tedious process, given what a person's assumptions are and how willing they are to listen. The outcome of not saying anything, however, is a guarantee that an autistic person will not learn. This will not likely cover every situation. Autistic people do by practice what most people know by instinct, so errors are always more probable, but patient explanation that avoids judgment could help minimize problems.

Then there are cases where relationships have been established. When an autistic person is in a relationship, they can experience communication issues that are unusual to most couples, although they can be solved.

Some forms of neurotypical interaction with their partner can be amusing. John Elder Robison, an autistic savant and author of *Look Me in the Eye* and other books, nicknamed his late ex-wife Unit Two (which she embraced) as well as her two sisters, which were Units One and Three, reflecting their birth order.[73]

Autistic people exhibit many positive qualities in relationships. They are famous for being unusually honest, both in their words and deeds. "My son is incapable of lying," said Ray Richmond, the father of an autistic son, age twenty-five, based in suburban Los Angeles.

In relationships, autistic people have also been known to have traits many people in society appreciate such as not being as overly concerned with appearance, less motivated by sexual desire, and more concerned with their partner's personality than neurotypicals tend to be, which helps them avoid some of the problems that may occur in neurotypical relationships.[74]

Like anyone else, autistic adults can also learn. Bruce Petherick, an Australian autistic musician and teacher now living in Alberta, Canada, learned how to handle a relationship through trial and error. He and his first wife gradually grew apart and eventually divorced. He was bewildered by his friends who had believed it was not going to work from the beginning but didn't tell him so before the wedding.

Petherick then met his second wife, who now helps raise his kids in Alberta. She is a social worker and was the person who led him to discover he was autistic. "It seems like I'm taking my work home with me," he described his then-girlfriend as having said. "It was watching *Big Bang Theory* and seeing Sheldon . . . it was 'that's exactly what I do, that's exactly what I do.'" After that assessment, which was well into adulthood, Petherick got diagnosed. Like many autistic people, he was relieved.

"I've been pretty successful as far as my professional life," he said. "But the painful aspects of my life could be attributed to my diagnosis." He alludes to struggles in general with being autistic, some of them deeply significant, that can also come into a marriage or relationship.

Some autistic people have routines and habits that their partner sees as strange or even repugnant, which need to be talked about to find a compromise. Some autistic partners may not be good at providing comfort in a way that neurotypical people often expect. This can make them frustrated when they're criticized for being uncaring.

A particularly common problem is that a neurotypical partner may also desire more affection and attention, while an autistic one may believe they are being too intrusive. This perhaps leads into discussing the most famous clinical book about autistic marriages, *Asperger's in Love* by therapist Maxine Aston, published in 2003.

Aston wrote the book based on stories from forty-one autistic people who fit the criteria for Asperger's syndrome before the autism spectrum was recognized by the DSM. She does discuss many positive aspects of autism in relationships, and though the autistic community would say some parts are too negative towards them, much of *Asperger's in Love* has credible advice for two people to manage their issues.

However, Aston made one major mistake that received a lot of attention that the autistic community viewed with contempt. She is credited with creating a concept called "Cassandra affective deprivation disorder," sometimes called "Cassandra syndrome."[75] Cassandra is a character in an ancient Greek myth who can tell the future, but no one believes her when she does, which causes her great pain. This metaphor is applied where communication difficulties exist between an autistic and neurotypical partner. This frustrates the neurotypical partner because they are not getting the affection they need and are unable to truly explain their needs and be believed.

While lack of showing affection can be an issue between neurotypical and autistic partners, just as with other couples, the idea of a psychiatric condition called "Cassandra syndrome" is not validated by current psychiatric literature.[76] There is also a good argument to be made that it is harmful as it heightens the likelihood that autistic people will be avoided as potential partners.

A fixation on concepts like Cassandra syndrome also ignores the possibility that an autistic person may have legitimate grievances against a neurotypical partner. Maybe they are pushing the autistic partner beyond their limits and in ways that are not constructive.

Additionally, the idea that neurotypical partners are inherently unhappy because they miss affection from their autistic spouses lacks a great deal of context. Autistic people are more likely to be sensitive to touch than neurotypicals, and they may want to be alone more often than neurotypicals. Some of them may manage with less sex than their neurotypical partner may like. This is not because of a lack of affection or real love from their partner; this may just reflect their own tolerance level for certain kinds of stimulation. To frame this another way, men typically have higher libidos than women, but women's lower sex drives (on average) are not usually framed as part of a disorder.[77]

There is a much simpler explanation for what the Cassandra syndrome attempts to explain: two people have not worked out their issues. Autistic people sometimes have issues as much as other people. They may need to communicate that and compromise with their partner. A neurotypical partner may prefer more outings in public than an autistic person likes. Or they may be annoyed with how their autistic partner communicates with others. This is a problem for two partners to work out like mature adults often must in a marriage.

The risk of an idea like Cassandra syndrome is it can scare neurotypical partners away from dating autistic people. This is potentially tragic given that they may find a great match, that all couples must work out issues, and the only difference is that an autistic person's issues are sometimes different in kind and scale to those of a neurotypical.

*Direct communication can be useful in any relationship, but it is often essential in relationships with autistic people.* There is potential for defensiveness and hurt feelings, as there would be for neurotypicals. But autistic people often have issues figuring out the intentions of others. If these are not communicated explicitly, they will not understand what they have done wrong or what they can do. In their experience, asking what they have done wrong can mean befuddlement from neurotypicals, and potential embarrassment and ridicule, so they may be much less likely to ask.

However, Petherick's story shows that a person who knows who they are and tailors their communication needs to their partner can do as well as any neurotypical couple. This sense of discovery might come later and with more obstacles than many neurotypicals, but Petherick shows that optimistic conclusions are possible. "I'm a very happy autistic person," he said.

## Online Communication

Even for autistic people who do not require AAC in ordinary daily life, changes in technology have made interaction easier, particularly online. A survey of autistic people showed that email was their most popular form of communication.[78] It can also come with side effects.

Online dating, for example, has made it easier and more comfortable for autistic people to find others. There is not much hard data on how many autistic people are online or how they compare to neurotypicals, but many like and even prefer dating online. This makes sense when someone understands an autistic person's characteristics.

Making initial moves when dating is full of complexity even for neurotypical people. Approaching someone they like requires an understanding of a lot of social cues. Are they with friends? Are they looking at them and showing interest non-verbally? How do they find out if they are in a relationship without seeming creepy? How fast do they go from casual introduction, to asking on a date, to engaging sexually? Deciphering and understanding this can provoke anxiety for anyone, and much more so for autistic people.

This all becomes much easier online.[79] Their friends are irrelevant when they first approach them. They are on the site and therefore want to be approached, and they are probably not in a relationship if they are on a dating site. Profile information also lets them know if they have common interests. It would be a bit like going into a bar where everyone's essential biography and current life state is floating over their head in a visible bubble. Such a world would make approaching someone much easier and lessen rejection.

There are also dangers. Some people online are predators or are at least not who they say they are (though this is also true of real life). Picking up on warning signs can be more difficult for an autistic person. Some of this risk can be mitigated through insisting on a video chat before meeting in person, which can usually confirm whether the person is basically who they described online. Getting to know them through an exclusively online relationship over a longer period before meeting in person may also mitigate risks.

For autistic women, who are especially vulnerable to men who may be looking for a hook-up or could even be a predator, this is a particular risk. They may also be more vulnerable because they lack social understanding and the confidence necessary to resist predatory behaviour and are even more likely to have issues with anxiety and depression. A trusted friend or family member can be a good person to ask for advice and support, which helps minimize the chance of being a victim of predators.

Starting up a conversation also happens more naturally, from an autistic perspective. A man can send a message to a woman and understands she will likely not respond right away, unlike during an in-person social setting. There are no facial expressions to decode, and there is plenty of time to comprehend the ebb and flow of the conversation.

Autistic people can also use this technology to make friends. For people who have strong interests, like many autistic people, meeting friends online can be easier when there is a barrier, namely the person's profile page, which shows they have something in common. Apart from autistic-specific dating apps like Hiki, websites like meetup.com allow autistic people to connect based on shared interests, which is an important way of bonding for many of them. This can also connect autistic and non-autistic people together.

During the wave of autistic-led organizations that started in the early 2000s, websites like wrongplanet.com, a forum founded by autistic teenager Alex Planck that allows autistic people to connect, started to emerge. That site was revolutionary for its time, and this ability to connect people continues today in the form of many websites like autismforum.com and the comments on popular autistic-created YouTube channels like The Aspie World, Asperger's from the Inside, Yo Samdy Sam, or Stephany Bethany, where autistic people can contact each other through comments sections and live chat sections. These are autistic people who give insight and information about the condition on their platforms and have communities of subscribers who can talk to each other and are popular among autistic people looking to relate to others.

During the COVID-19 pandemic, the use of online connection on platforms like Zoom changed everyone's lives. It became essential to people working from home, and it also meant events that would previously have been held in person became hosted online. This has been received especially positively in the autism world. Zoom does not require looking other people in the eye or even seeing or hearing the other person, as in-person conversation often does, because of the chat feature. It does not even require going into public places where sensory issues may cause problems with attention and focus, and autistic people may be more likely to feel safe and protected, especially when meeting strangers.

This does not mean autistic people should restrict themselves to online communication. Physical connection is ultimately a necessity for all people, but this technology offers another way to start a connection that is less intimidating for many autistic people. That is a victory.

Many autistic adults see the advent of the internet as a generally positive development. The opportunities offered are new; the negative aspects mimic the real world in ways that are not pleasant but have always been there.

*Neurotypical people can also help autistic people in their lives understand the subtleties of online communication that may be missed.* They more readily understand the complex social cues involved in dating and can be good mentors to help autistic people be themselves while also understanding others.

When it's used right, technology can facilitate communication for a group of people whose lives have seldom been easy. This results in decreased anxiety, which also makes it easier for autistic people to show the sides of themselves they most like.

## Positive Traits of Autistic Communication

The challenges autistic people have with communication are well-known. Many autistic people would say, however, that there are positive sides to the way they communicate of which they are quite proud and grateful.

Ilana Garvey (not her real name), a young woman from the United States, said she learned early on to be herself and not let the opinions of others bother her. Many autistic people are deeply wounded by negative opinions of them. For others, learning not to let this bother them is a common lesson taken even early in life, one which many neurotypicals are never forced to learn as starkly. She said:

> I didn't care about social norms, I didn't care what other people thought. I'd also heard in anti-bullying PSAs that bullies only bully because they're insecure or hurt etc., and while I think many bullying victims didn't believe that (at least that I spoke to/was friends with), I just took it literally. So, when someone bullied me, I just saw it as invalid, that it didn't mean anything.

Autistic people are known for being intensely honest. This can cause social problems because the honesty can be the same when they tell their spouse their clothes make them look fat and when they are testifying in court. It can also lead to a tendency to overshare personal information.

"I can come across as a little abrupt," said Jacob Dean, a young autistic man studying to be a general practitioner in England. "I don't mean to, but I can offend people as well. That's just me saying what's on my mind without filtering it."

There is, however, another side. Honesty is also a classic virtue. One positive aspect of this is that autistic people are not known for having "hidden agendas." If an autistic person tells someone they are okay, they really are likely okay. If an autistic person tells someone they were somewhere, they may misremember or get confused, especially under stress, but they are probably not consciously lying. They are often not trying to hide something. Even when an autistic person tries to lie, it is less likely to be successful.[80]

This lack of deception can also extend to their personalities. Though many autistic people "mask" certain traits to fit into a neurotypical group, and other people do not mention their own problems, some proudly say they do not hide themselves. "I think it's a disability to always live in a mask and pretend you're somebody you're not," said M., who went on to tell a story about a conference she attended where the presenter said that everyone had a "social mask." "That sounds so alien to me, it's just 'who you see is who I am.'"

Apart from the general tendency to be honest, there are other advantages to being unabashedly autistic. Michael John Carley, who grew up when modern autism diagnosis was not possible, also said when he was a teenager and was being abused in school that his combative personality helped him. He said this hurt him in the short term and "made life miserable" for his mother but helped him psychologically because he did not hide his troubles. "I hadn't felt like a victim all through those years because I stood up for myself," he said during an appearance on the *Uniquely Human* podcast. "There was some punk thing that said, 'I don't like you either,' and I said so."[81] Carley also said that his combativeness helped him stave off potential predators, who otherwise would have seen him as an ideal target.

The odd paradox is that evidence suggests autistic people may be seen as deceptive by neurotypicals because of what are seen as odd ways autistic people present themselves socially. They are less likely to look someone in the eye, and they are more likely to fidget, which can make them appear deceptive, but this is more likely a sign of anxiety than lying.[82]

Despite appearances though, the honesty is still there. For those who know autistic people well, it can be refreshing. They don't have to wonder what the autistic person in their life is really thinking.

Their honesty and commitment can also extend to morality. Although this area still needs more study, researchers at Middlesex University in England hypothesized that autistic traits may make a person more likely to be a whistleblower within their workplace.[83] Because autistic people can have a rigid set of moral rules, which are somewhat innate and somewhat learned, their purpose as moral agents can be to apply them absolutely.[84]

This becomes a communication issue because the intentions behind such a rigid set of rules can end up being misunderstood. It can also make the person living by that code, including telling superiors when it's broken, unpopular. Unsurprisingly, this is especially true among the people they are informing on, particularly starting in adolescence. "It's one thing to rat on people in elementary school," said Todd Simkover, a self-employed autistic self-advocate reflecting on his experiences as a child. "When you rat out the wrong people in high school, [it can cause a problem]."

Even autistic children are more apt to report someone they think has broken rules. However, when reported on themselves, they are more likely to complain about the facts of the incident in question rather than focus on the betrayal and the person informing on them.[85] An autistic person may sometimes have to learn that there is a difference between telling to get someone into trouble and telling to prevent someone from doing harm, but there is a virtue to putting principles above social niceties.

At an abstract personal level, an autistic friend may not be the person to confess an affair to if the goal is to keep it secret and get non-judgmental reassurance. But is reassurance always the right response? An autistic person may be (and probably is) right about the friend being in the wrong. It is also a genuine question whether keeping that secret from the spouse works in the couple's best long-term interests.

Of course, a neurotypical can have the same train of thought, but autistic people are likely to think about these questions more starkly and automatically, and in a black-and-white moral context.[86] These judgments can be appropriate, or they may not fit the situation, just as loyalty to friends and not revealing their activities can either be a sign of compassion and understanding or part of a criminal cover-up. This tendency by autistic people should not be mistaken for a lack of loyalty. They can be extremely reliable and dedicated friends — it just doesn't usually come at the expense of the truth or the rules.

Of course, neurotypicals can see a greater good than personal loyalty, and some cultures view personal loyalty as a more important value than other cultures. However, this instinct comes more immediately to autistic people. If the scenario is a company defrauding customers, an autistic person blowing the whistle is the person most likely to be commended in that scenario.[87]

There are multiple possible reasons for this attitude towards morality. Autistic people are particularly anxious in the face of change and ambiguity. Just like with changing routines or living spaces, not following the rules can create intense discomfort. The world stops becoming predictable, which can leave an autistic person in a state of chaos. Correcting moral wrongs can help set their own world right.

There is a more noble reason, which has to do with setting *the world* right. It is impossible to right every wrong, but having a strong moral code that is difficult to shake can be a good trait in and of itself. While moral rules sometimes have exceptions, as two principles can sometimes conflict with each other, there is also a significant problem of making moral issues too flexible. To use an old aphorism showing both points of view, "the branch that doesn't bend, breaks," but "bend too far, and you're already broken."

This categorical thinking can also lead to acts of altruism that would not be immediately thought of by many neurotypical people. An act like whistleblowing involves a lot of personal courage and sacrifice, which can often be justified if the principle is that important and the action that clearly wrong.

This black-and-white thinking can motivate autistic people to give a lot of money to help someone in need. A study by Uta and Chris Frith also suggests that they give the same amount even if someone else is not looking, which indicates they are motivated by the principle of generosity itself.[88]

This is not to suggest autistic people are incorruptible paragons of virtue. Autistic people have all the same moral temptations and frailties as anyone else. They need love, connection, security, status, and the means to survive. They can be pushed to hurt others or take their property if they do not get it, just like anyone else. They commit crimes at rates no higher than the general population but are capable of criminality.[89]

Nevertheless, there are traits that can be more evident in autistic people that can make them good to have in other's lives: self-assurance, honesty, dedication, lack of pretense, and strong fundamental moral principles. Many neurotypicals are often taken aback by some of the seemingly naïve ways autistic people interact with others; they may not consider their other positive aspects, which may emerge later once they start to get to know them.

As a practical matter, this should be considered when autistic people are in a social setting. *Ask an autistic person why they think something, rather than dismiss it. If the explanation isn't satisfying, explain why.*

*But also, don't pooh-pooh an autistic person's point of view automatically.* They will make social mistakes and may give advice that if followed would be a disaster. This comes from a certain understanding of the world that may not make sense in some contexts but may contain a grain of truth.

Autistic and neurotypical people alike are sometimes keen to make quick judgments. It takes patient communication to really understand a person, in all their human strengths and frailties.

## Conclusion

Issues with social communication can do a lot to make an autistic person feel alien. With enough effort and understanding by both autistic and non-autistic people, however, this feeling could be less and less impactful.

The good news about bridging differences between autistic and neurotypical communication is that neither person must learn a new language or gain any specialized knowledge, though some of the latter may help just for context.

What it really takes is patience, understanding, and willingness to listen, and most people are capable of that. For neurotypical people, this can be done in several ways.

- Understand how autistic people, particularly adults, see the social world.
- If it becomes evident that a person may be autistic, it becomes especially important to take your time and apply this understanding.
- If this autistic person is someone a neurotypical cares for, provide them what they need to communicate, including AAC if needed.
- Be especially careful not to get too loud, animated, or unpredictable, as autistic people are more likely to freak out.
- Always try to see their side of a disagreement, even if the explanation may seem odd, because it isn't likely to be odd to them.
- Be willing to negotiate any disagreements and explain how a neurotypical sees the world as well.

Like any kind of disability, autism often makes people interact with the world more slowly and deliberately. A person on crutches or a wheelchair will not be as fast as a person on foot, and an autistic person will not process social communication as quickly or accurately as a neurotypical.

To take the analysis to a more abstract level, it could help to imagine a world where autistic social communication is the norm for most human beings. It would almost certainly rely on direct speech, rather than metaphor and non-verbal cues. It would likely prioritize truth over personal feelings. It may be a little more emotionally volatile, as emotional regulation can be an issue, though it may not result in as many long-term grudges. It may involve more judgment of actions but less prejudice of appearance.

It may not be a better world, especially for neurotypicals. However, it is useful to imagine considering autism as a different culture instead of a defect, but also for them to imagine what it is like to be in a world they do not instinctively understand.

Neurotypical journalists who have written about autism and been in predominantly autistic places have sometimes come away with a different view of the world. This was Steve Silberman's take-away from going to Autreat, an autistic-run conference last held in 2013 that was organized by Autism Network International.

> My conversations at Autreat — some mediated by keyboards or other devices for augmenting communication — taught me more about the day-to-day realities of being autistic than reading a hundred case studies would. They also offered me the chance to be in the neurological minority for the first time in my life, which illuminated some of the challenges that autistic people face in a society not built for them, while disabusing me of pernicious stereotypes such as the idea that autistic people lack humour or creative imagination. After just four days in autismland, the mainstream world seemed like a constant sensory assault.[90]

Autreat was also famous for its "Ask a Neurotypical" forum, where autistic people would be able to ask neurotypicals on a stage about the way they see the world and compare it to themselves.[91] The aim of this was always to avoid condescension or bullying. It was sincerely meant as a way for two different brain types to understand each other. This kind of mutual understanding is what is needed more often, both for the sake of neurotypicals and autistic people, especially when it comes to communication issues.

At the end of his account, Silberman alludes to sensory issues as part of this culture. This is not a communication issue but instead deals with the other, and equally significant, diagnostic category shared by all autistic people.

## CHAPTER 4:
## RESTRICTED AND REPETITIVE BEHAVIOURS

THE SECOND DSM-5 CRITERIA FOR AUTISM are restricted or repetitive behaviours. The subcategories recognized in the DSM are repeated activities, strict routines, intense interests, and issues with the sensory environment. These sensory issues can include sounds being too loud, sights being too bright, or tastes being too intense.

Though these traits are so common in autistic people that they are used to diagnose autism more broadly, there is an underlying logic to why autistic people have them. Even though these behaviours are often more visible, extreme, and socially unacceptable to enough people to make life harder for autistic people when exhibiting them, what they are doing is fundamentally based on feelings all human beings have: they are trying to create a sense of control out of chaos.

As autistic self-advocate Theresa Jolliffe put it:

> Reality to an autistic person is a confusing interacting mass of events, people, places, sounds, and sights. There seems to be no clear boundaries, order, or meaning to anything. A large part of my life is spent trying to work out the pattern behind everything.[1]

Just as autistic people make rigid rules to deal with the chaos of social communication, they also classify things into rigid categories to make sense of the world. Because this process is learned rather than intuitive, and because these rules can sometimes be learned wrong, like any skill, how autistic people behave can look unnatural and bizarre to neurotypicals.

What neurotypicals may not realize is that autistic people are often behaving in a way that reflects how they've understood the world. They are not built with an intuitive comprehension of how the world works that others share, so they must create it themselves with a lot of practice and observation. Think of it as trying to glue together a broken vase without ever having even seen a picture of one. Sometimes there isn't even an intuitive understanding of the final goal. Eventually, you may come up with a workable estimation, but it takes time and a lot of trial and error.

To autistic people, others do not make sense, social structures do not make sense, and the physical world humans create can often be disorienting and without structures to lessen this. When you understand life from that perspective, autistic people's behaviour almost always makes much more sense. They are trying their best to operate in the world.

When autistic people cannot use these coping mechanisms or engage in some of these behaviours, it can lead to intense frustration. If it overflows, it can lead to meltdowns or shutdowns. Meltdowns are when they release all these feelings through a strong emotional reaction, like a shouting spurt. Shutdowns are when they withdraw and stay quiet, shutting out the world. Both are temporary, lasting from minutes to hours, though their exact length varies depending on the circumstances.[2]

These are almost always unpleasant experiences for autistic people. They are also behaviours that are easier to explain to neurotypicals as many can imagine what it is like to be overwhelmed to the point of tears or screaming. What makes autism different is the triggers for these meltdowns and shutdowns. They can include events neurotypical people barely notice, which go unfiltered by a sense of chaos and an overactive sensory system.[3]

As with neurotypicals, meltdowns and shutdowns can be more frequent in childhood, though they happen at all ages. In adults, they may become less prevalent as people learn to manage their emotions and orient the world in a way that is less confusing.[4]

However, autistic adults are still autistic, which means that in some conditions they will find the world overwhelming in ways that their peers, and even people younger than them, will likely not. Regulating emotions is always a struggle for autistic people at any age.

No matter how much an autistic person learns, the world will never completely make sense like it will to a neurotypical, in the same way a long-time foreigner may speak the language in another culture but always have an accent.

Other restricted and repetitive behaviours are not solely coping mechanisms for a chaotic world. Some of the criteria reflected in the DSM are motivated by activities giving them joy and comfort, regardless of the person's environment. These traits, in some contexts, can even have positive impacts on their development, including inspiring pursuit of hobbies that provide them with purpose and connection. Their intense level of focus, in some cases, can give them the practice needed to do something well.

## Special Interests/Passions

Special interests, as clinicians have historically called them, or passions, as more autistic people call them, are one of the most enjoyable parts of life for many people on the spectrum.[5] These intense personal interests can be directed at various topics that can often take up a disproportionate amount of focus and attention in an autistic person's life.

These passions are among the more common traits, involving 75% to 95% of autistic people, and are some of the earliest observed.[6] Both Kanner and Asperger saw this in the kids they described in their earliest papers and came to two different conclusions.

Kanner took a dim view of these interests, calling the ability to pick up names and facts the result of an "excellent rote memory, coupled with the inability to use rote language in any other way." He also believed children's use of language in memorizing details cut into general language development.[7]

Asperger, by contrast, believed some of these interests reflected genuine talents. He also noticed that information about these interests was acquired through personal motivation, not through outside pressure, which makes such learning second nature.

> Another autistic child had specialized technological interests and knew an incredible amount about complex machinery. He acquired this knowledge through constant questioning, which it was impossible to fend off, and to a great degree through his own observations.[8]

Asperger treated multiple children like this at Heilpädagogik, including a fifteen-year-old who was so absorbed in an interest in chemistry that he stole chemistry equipment from his school.[9] He also wrote about one patient who later went on to become an assistant professor in astronomy, showing that autistic people have potential to apply their interests with the right support.[10]

What is believed about passions now? It's complicated, but the general view is probably more Aspergian than Kannerian. Passions provide a great deal of pleasure for autistic people and should be treated largely like a neurotypical's passionate hobby. *Let them enjoy and develop them.* It often gives them joy, and it can even give them purpose and a source of work if it is properly nurtured. It can also help develop life skills.

"Politics helps me realize things aren't black and white," said Brianna Callanan, an autistic woman in her twenties from Massachusetts, talking about how this interest allows her to see multiple sides of an issue, which increases awareness of others.

While they should be treated the same, neurotypical hobbies and special interests are different. What usually distinguishes a special interest from a neurotypical interest is its intensity, purpose, and expression.[11]

In children, these interests may focus on extremely narrow details, like garage door openers or camera models, without any interest in houses or photography in general.[12] In adults, these pursuits can still be narrow but tend to broaden to some degree.[13] These can also increase in number and sophistication, as they become more and more exposed to subjects that may interest them, which can make conversations easier as their world expands.[14]

These activities frequently centre on things, rather than people, but not always. This tendency makes autistic people disproportionately involved in science, technology, math, and engineering (STEM). In addition to being really dedicated collectors and avid readers, they may be interested in philosophy, literature, games, music, history, and other subjects outside of STEM.[15] This is an example of how a stereotype can reflect real trends but should not be applied to individuals.

This specialized and intense interest can lead to remarkable expertise in their subject. As anecdotal evidence, Ray Richmond, who lives in the greater Los Angeles area, sees this ability in his son who is in his mid-twenties. "He's incredibly able to focus intently," he said. "He can hyperfocus on things and particularly on music, in audio engineering . . . to the point where he doesn't really want to be involved in anything else."

Employers may praise autistic adults for the extent of their job-related technical expertise. As one survey shows, of all the issues that autistic people face at work, excessive work demands were not generally seen as a problem. To the contrary, *lack* of challenge on the job sometimes was seen as a problem.[16]

Autistic people can also have talents that match these interests. A higher-than-average number are believed to have a trait called hyperlexia, the ability to read and write before the age of five or six, when children are normally expected to learn to read.[17] This allows autistic people to sound out more advanced books at an earlier age and helps them to do better in school. There is sometimes a lack of true understanding of what they are reading, even though they can sound it out from an early age, but it is nevertheless a powerful skill for many with this trait.[18]

What these interests all provide is joy and relief from anxiety because they are predictable and a source of intrinsic pleasure. They can even help an autistic person get through life. For Thomas Yackimec, an autistic man in his mid-twenties from northern Alberta, his passion for music was the only motive for him to attend school. "High school, I didn't really care too much for because I felt stifled a little bit," he said. "The only thing that kind of kept me interested was music half the time, which is the only reason I bothered to study at all." He later studied music at Grant MacEwan College in Edmonton and now composes music while also working for Alberta Parks. His earlier struggles with school are common for autistic people. Unfortunately, having an outlet that salvaged school is less common.

Some overall gender differences in interests are also suspected. Females have been observed to have more of an interest in animals, fiction, and fantasy than males, though of course this is not absolute.[19] "I still like to collect children's books," said Sudhanshu Grover. "I still read them. . . . If I cannot buy them, I will look them up on YouTube and listen to the stories. . . . I'm also a big-time *Star Wars* and Marvel fan."

Anyone who has been to any gaming or sci-fi convention knows there is also plenty of overlap in Grover's interests with men. Special interests/passions are as variable as the condition of autism itself. The combinations can be endless.

However, some pursuits seem to be gender specific. For instance, adolescent and adult females have been observed having traditional young girl interests, such as Barbies. Though, the way they express this interest can be unusual, such as having a larger collection of Barbies, categorizing them unconventionally, not part of playtime with friends.[20]

This is much like a boy who expresses his interest in sports by collecting thousands of playing cards and memorizing statistics rather than involving his friends with them. This way of undertaking interests, namely collecting experiences or things, can also extend into adulthood. It is often a source of pleasure and accomplishment.

However, there are some downsides to the expression of these passions. Other people may think it's boring and annoying when autistic people get so wrapped up in talking about their subject. The lack of reciprocal interest by others can make it seem like they only care about themselves, which is not usually the truth. The autistic person is often just reflecting their passion, as well as a desire to keep the world predictable by talking about things they know.

Therefore, it is important to let autistic people talk about their interests. This gives them a sense of stability and peace.

Nevertheless, if the disconnect between a neurotypical and an autistic person carries on long enough, this can cause friction.[21] Because the expression of these interests can potentially isolate autistic people from others, this can also be the basis of bullying in childhood and possible rejection, withdrawal, and self-consciousness as an adult. While this often says more about the morals of those doing the bullying and rejecting, the likelihood of this rejection is nevertheless a disadvantage.

There is also no guarantee that autistic people will excel, even in their subject of interest, as some people may assume. Although this ability to excel is true of some, there is a wider range of academic achievement among autistic people: some do better or much better than average and others don't do well at all. Overall, while the extremes can be more populated by autistic people, as a whole they perform about as well as neurotypicals.[22]

However, the sensory environment, the way the subject is framed and taught, the social lives of autistic people, and other factors can override even a passionate interest.[23] When at its most intense, the interest can also distract from more productive activities, which autistic people need to do to take care of themselves.[24] In more highly unusual circumstances, its pull can lead to dangerous, antisocial, or illegal behaviour. Even in these cases, something deeper than the interest itself may cause this behaviour.

Something beneath the surface can reveal profound insight into autistic people's talents, and the opportunities they are not being afforded. One of the most famous cases is that of Darius McCollum, an autistic New Yorker whose passion was the New York City transit system. Over the last few decades, he has done multiple stints in jail for hijacking subways and buses. He did this while also being rejected for a job at the greater New York area's Metropolitan Transit Authority, despite applying numerous times.

McCollum has become a folk hero in some autistic circles because the motive for doing this was at no time malicious. He never harmed his passengers, he never hijacked vehicles to make demands, and those he hijacked sometimes even made their scheduled stops. His motive was a desire to work in the world of transit, and his lack of ability to achieve this made him feel the need to do so illegally.[25]

This ultimate motive shows the sheer scale of the joy that autistic people can get from their passions. The analogy that best explains the quality of a special interest to neurotypicals is by comparing it to falling in love. The passion is there; the variety of its expression can be as well.

The passion can be a blip of time and then change to something else, or it can last an autistic person's entire life. It can be rationally based in certain other connected aspects of their personality, or it can be irrational and inexplicable. They can have one or multiple at any time.[26]

What usually never changes is the feeling of engaging in these subjects. When an autistic person gets really interested in a topic, the preoccupation with it can be called obsessive by some, passion-filled by others, but fundamentally it is an experience like developing a deep relationship with someone.

The analogy of love continues in that most neurotypicals understand the initial infatuation and interest when a person first meets the love of their life, gets married, or has a child. It is more common at these high points for neurotypical people to behave in a way that is "autistic-like." They talk about the person or their child frequently to their friends, they can act in ways that are "mushy" and annoying to others, and many neurotypical people can even relate to those who commit a crime for a person that they love or rob a bank to feed their family. It's not unlike McCollum risking prison to feed his love of transit.

These are ultimately relatable experiences to most people, and therefore are excused and not stigmatized. That same level of understanding is often not applied to autistic interests, and neurotypicals commonly see the same way of expression in this context as socially odd.

Of course, it is unreasonable to expect to live in a world where illegal behaviour can be assumed to be rewarded. But a story like McCollum's provokes two questions: What barriers prevent someone like him, who perhaps knew more about the New York City transit system than most of its employees, from being a productive person in society? And why can't more autistic people use their passions to get into productive careers?

Later in this book, some barriers are explored in more detail that make it difficult for autistic people to get employment in areas of interest that are meaningful to them. Challenges for autistic people in the education system, which can be significant for some, or in maintaining employment because of social skills issues or sensory issues, can mean that many miss out on opportunities available to people without their challenges.

A wide-ranging knowledge of autism, even more than the remarkable changes in public attitudes since Lorna Wing's spectrum became mainstream, would assist others to properly understand autistic people's behaviours. Help can be provided where necessary for the people-related and sensory aspects of work, including with reasonable accommodations, that can reveal their talents and expertise.

There is also an impracticality that can result from an autistic person's special interest. If the passion is narrow enough, it can be difficult to form a career out of it. What some people don't consider, however, is that the interest is worthwhile even if it does not lead to a career, just as a neurotypical person's hobby does not have to be monetized to be beneficial to them.

Passions are one of the best aspects of having autism. They offer a sense of security because engaging with interests is much more predictable than dealing with people. They provide an excuse to recover from a chaotic environment. They also afford a sense of purpose that comes from within them, which is often the most meaningful part of life.

*Because of this, autistic people with unique interests and talents must be encouraged to pursue them, whether as hobbies or at work. Neurotypical employers should always consider the talents and especially the passion of autistic people.*

These are people who have a lot to offer under the right circumstances. It can be as little as great conversation material — autistic people can be full of fascinating information if others are willing to listen.

Interests can also lead to the development of something practical and even career-building, but the stakes here are significant. Being underemployed or unemployed makes it more likely that any adult will be depressed, insecure, dependent, and anxious. Autistic adults are no exception. The question of autistic people using their passions relates to their own quality of life, and even the health of the entire society.

Fulfillment can also come from sources other than employment and can be something that gives meaning to life. For a group of people with passions and motivations, sharing these interests is just one way that autistic adults can live more fulfilling lives.

## Routines

If special interests are one of the more pleasurable autistic traits, routines are among the most classic.

In his 1943 paper, Leo Kanner wrote that Donald Triplett got deeply upset when his routine was disrupted. This even went as far as repeating the same action again and again.

> Most of his actions were repetitions carried out exactly the same way in which they had been performed originally. If he spun a block, he must always start with the same face uppermost. When he threaded buttons, he arranged them in a certain sequence that had no pattern to it but happened to be the order used by his father when he first showed them to Donald.[27]

Of course, many people like familiarity and have routines to keep their lives in order. It's even considered part of a healthy and productive way of living life. But as with passions, what is different for many autistic people is the extent these are part of their lives and their consistency and rigidity.

They take the same route to work and find it distressing to take a detour. Other autistic people watch a certain TV show at the same time every single day. Others have the exact same food for breakfast, lunch, or dinner at the same time and get distressed when their routine is disrupted. Some only like seeing certain people at certain times.[28]

This level of sameness is not common among neurotypicals; most would consider this kind of routine a form of oppression. The oddity of autistic routines from a neurotypical point of view was parodied in a sketch on the satire show *The Onion*, where an autistic reporter demands to be put in prison when he hears about its highly structured and rigid daily routine from a prisoner.[29] This is a comic exaggeration, of course, but it is insightful in how it shows the motive for this degree of routine. As covered from the outset, this is a way of making sense of a senseless world.

Ilana Garvey related:

> For [the last] eight to nine years or so, I've taken the exact same bike route. I put on music and take the same route every time. I love it because I can focus on the sensory experience of biking — the wind, the vestibular sensation, the proprioceptive sensation of the movements, my music — and let my imagination wander without having to focus on which way to go.
>
> I've had roughly the same morning routine for years with small tweaks as life changes. I reread the same books all the time — and genuinely enjoy them. New books are great too, but there's something about the familiarity of a book that you've read ten times before and the characters you love that's soothing. And I still get excited for my favorite parts. It's satisfying to see the characters succeed, even though I knew it would happen. The same goes for TV shows and movies.

Garvey's anecdote also shows a fact that can sometimes be overlooked if viewed too much through stereotypes. The level and rigidity of the routines can differ among autistic people. Some may just like the same food every day at certain meals and are otherwise flexible, while others meticulously manage every aspect of their lives.

Just because someone is autistic does not mean it is the end of the world to change plans. It may just be a matter of which plans to alter and how much notice and care is given in doing so. How to handle changes in routine is different from person to person.

When they don't change, however, these tendencies can be frustrating for neurotypicals and harmful to autistic people. One example from the clinical literature is an autistic man who wore the same ripped shirt and boxers to bed and insisted on this even on his honeymoon. He did this simply because that was what he wore to bed normally and didn't want to change. Let's just say, his wife was not happy.[30]

This story extends beyond not following the latest fashions, which autistic people have also been known for.[31] It also shows how sometimes their routines can become pathological, including when they involve not washing themselves properly or insist other people in their lives conform to what they do.

This rigidity can hurt autistic people in relationships with friends and romantic partners and in the workplace. It is one thing to have an inflexible routine that makes a person feel comfortable, but routines can sometimes extend to not wanting to quit a job and look for a better one. They can involve not moving out of their parents' house even when they can, or not giving up a certain hobby or friend even when it impinges on their well-being. For some more obviously autistic people, getting them to change a routine might be especially difficult.

Anyone can struggle with these aspects of adult life, but they can become more extreme and entrenched in autistic people who have made these routines a part of their lives. It is moments like these that indicate when change is clearly necessary, and how not changing them shows just how important it can be for them to feel in control. A change can make an autistic person slip into chaos, which to them can be worse than mediocrity.

Some routines don't hurt other people, and they make autistic people comfortable. *These routines should not be touched.* For those that are a problem, compromises are sometimes possible to help autistic adults tailor their routines towards not impacting others. It may involve some tactful negotiation and maybe some arguments, but autistic people are not immune to reason and often can listen. If a routine is hurting someone in their life, and that can be clearly communicated, many will think about changing, as difficult as this may be for them.

There are also ways to help an autistic person use this tendency to their advantage and use it to get them on a path that will satisfy them long-term. Starting in the 1960s, it became obvious to educators that structured routines should be part of the way autistic people stay oriented and learn. A commonly used form of Eric Schopler's TEACCH program, founded in 1972, is called structured teaching.[32] Its backbone is highly structured surroundings, such as plants always being in the right place in the classroom, but also a highly structured and scheduled routine.

This is an example of one such program for autistic students in early adolescence.[33]

8:30 – Student arrival, put belongings away, greetings
8:45 – Work session 1
9:30 – Work session 2

10:15 – Break
10:30 – Leisure learning/school friends
11:00 – Work session 3
11:45 – Prepare for lunch
12:00 – Lunch
12:30 – Outside/gym
1:00 – Clean cafeteria tables and floors
1:45 – Work session 4
2:30 – Dismissal

TEACCH also has programs for autistic adults based on their principles. They have unemployment services, an internship training program, post-secondary school help, and a residential service centre called the Carolina Living and Service Centre.[34]

If this program resembles a regular school day, except slightly more regimented, it's because structure is often beneficial for all children and adults, not just autistic ones.[35] Getting into a habit where people establish time for themselves to achieve what they want sets up long-term success.[36] This can be applied to both a person who is single-mindedly focused on their career or someone who plans out their day for a nine-to-five job with evenings to socialize. If something is important, making time for it through structure is beneficial.

Questions of routine also inevitably bring up questions of time management, which involves perceptions of time to begin with. When autistic people are not adhering to their routines, they are more likely to get overwhelmed and lose their sense of time. Some evidence suggests autistic children and adolescents have issues with temporal processing. This is done by the part of the brain that also controls much of the auditory system. This trait of being able to process time is linked with life outcome measures, and problems with it are sometimes compensated for by having alarms and a schedule, or by bribing oneself.

For example, a study among nine- to seventeen-year-olds measured their ability to tell when four, eight, twelve, sixteen, or twenty seconds had passed. Impairments with this system are considered a classic trait of ADHD, which autistic people are more likely to have than the general population.[37] With autistic people in general, independent of ADHD, the jury is still out on whether temporal processing is a core deficit, but time management has been observed in clinical studies to be an issue.

Some autistic people have difficulty determining what is important in a project and setting a dedicated amount of time to it that is reasonable and effective to complete the job.[38] They may base this amount on how much it attracts their attention or interest, and sometimes they can get bored if it does not.

However, autistic people have a contradiction in this way that people with ADHD do not. Employers in Australia, according to one study, have reported their autistic employees are generally reliable at work and arrive on time.[39] Autistic people can be very punctual, expect punctuality from others, and can get frustrated when something does not go as expected.

On a very preliminary basis, this difference might be explained by their routines, which help establish autistic people in a predictable world and make sense of how it operates. These are critical for people who have difficulty with chaos.

*As a general rule, autistic adults should have their routines respected unless there is a deeply compelling reason not to, such as a risk to their short- or long-term health.* If they insist on taking a specific route to their job, for example, let them enjoy their route.

Without the routines, they are literally lost in time. "Empty time," as Lillian Burke of the Redpath Centre in Toronto has written about, is often a period where autistic people who are unsure of what to do show anxious behaviours.[40] These include one of autism's most visible, stigmatized, and misunderstood traits.

## Stimming

If there is an area of autism that has sometimes been most obvious, and sometimes most disturbing to those who do not understand autism, it may be the repetitive behaviours autistic people use to help calm themselves. These are called stims, and the action of using them is called stimming, which is short for "self-stimulation."

All humans stim. Whether the stim is tapping a foot or twiddling a pencil or fidget spinner, all people have physical ways of relieving stress and showing nervousness. Stimming in autism, however, is unique.

The biggest difference between autistic and neurotypical stimming is that autistic people do this more often and in ways that are more exuberant and noticeable to others. These stims are particularly stigmatized in people whose autism is more obvious. This can be violently rocking back and forth while shaking one's arms. This can be loud grunting noises. This can be talking very loudly to themselves, whether it is something going on in their mind or humming or parroting something they saw elsewhere. For people with less obvious autistic traits, this can include tapping that is louder, or humming audibly, or jumping up and down excitedly. Others engage in hobbies and play in a way that provides order and calms them down.

Ilana Garvey[41] describes her actions:

> I tap and flick my fingers, crack my knuckles . . . [I] chew on my lip, rub textures (e.g., the stitching on the armrest of a couch), bounce my feet, rub my feet together (especially when going to bed), etc. I only hand flap when I'm extremely excited, but there's that one too.
>
> When I was a kid, I was *very* repetitive in my imaginative play. I would take my Playmobil people on "journeys" and would literally line them up on horses and in wagons and move one, then the next, then the next in a line. I did the same with Hot Wheel cars on a car rug. I could play like that for *hours*. It was very imaginative, though. There was an entire story of why they were adventuring and how each character felt about what was happening.

For decades, clinicians have reported that autistic children lack imaginative play. Essentially, this means that rather than, for example, imagining dolls and action figures as their characters in play, they will sort them in patterns they notice. This is the kind of activity that Garvey is referring to. It is imaginative, just with a different kind of imagination.

What Garvey is doing is the same as what anyone else does when they are trying to relieve stress. The difference is that autistic stims are seen as weird, and often misunderstood. They can be perceived as the actions of a person that is undesirable and pitiable.

While stimming has been shown sometimes to interfere with learning — and in that context, there might be a reason to help autistic people reduce it — trying to stigmatize and seriously dissuade them in all circumstances is usually a mistake.[42]

Nevertheless, the apparent peculiarity of stimming has been used for propaganda purposes to show what a "menace" autism is. In 2002, a U.S. congressional hearing on vaccines and autism included a video of a young autistic boy walking around fidgeting with his hands and making noises. The implication was to show how autism is harmful.[43]

The premise of the hearing was wrong, in retrospect, as vaccines do not cause autism. Even more to the point is that the child shown is merely autistic, which for some neurotypicals is sufficiently unusual. While this child, who would now be an adult, likely struggles with many parts of life that neurotypicals do not, he was not sick and especially should not have been deemed to be based on his stimming.

The video also shows a lack of understanding on how stims, like many other aspects of autism, can change from childhood to adulthood. Some adults lose stims they had when they were younger, sometimes through therapy and training, covering it up to avoid humiliation, or through development.[44] This childhood stimming is not a sign of pathology to begin with, and while it might never completely stop, the person in the video may no longer present that way as an adult.

Stimming is also an area where elements of autism become integrated, and where different parts of the DSM are related to each other. Although it is often a response to sensory issues in the external environment, like reacting to bright lights, it can also come from inside a person's own head, such as thinking obsessively about something that happened to them or that they saw. In other words, these stims are highly context-dependent and more likely to occur in situations that are unusual or triggering.

This does not mean an autistic adult should be coddled and made to avoid any potentially uncomfortable situation. All humans must face these situations at some point in their lives, and this can be a source of growth.

But stimming can often indicate that they may be reaching their limits, and it is more productive to understand them this way compared to how they have historically been treated, which is to assume that these are bad or weird behaviours to be corrected.

There is a strong argument that this is more of a problem of society's perceptions rather than of the autistic person themselves. Stimming, at the very least, should not be punished, in children or adults. Most stims are not harmful and are often an outlet to manage strong emotions, which come with their condition.

This comes with one exception: the risk of self-injury for some autistic people. This can include headbanging and rubbing body parts against rough objects, scratching, biting, or pinching. These are the most worrying kinds. For children, these can help them get in touch with their bodies or gain attention from other people for their needs. They can also communicate a message to others in the absence of a healthier alternative.

Although this can also apply to autistic adults, there is the added component of self-harm related to depression and suicide. No link has been established between self-injurious stims in autistic people and suicidal behaviour, but their higher rates of depression mean that adult self-injury must be looked at as a possible warning sign, as it would be in anyone else.[45]

In some ways, self-harming stims can be relatable to neurotypical people. Some of them feel so overwhelmed that they will cut their bodies or even kill themselves. Those who do not experience these feelings are likely to have at least heard about such people.

Just like with non-injury stims, the subjective experience of such feelings is not different in how autistic people experience it; it's just that their thresholds and triggers for stress are different. Regardless of motive, these kinds of stims can be dangerous to the person using them and must be treated differently from non-injurious stims.

Self-injury is also related to a broader issue. Because stimming in general is linked to anxiety, efforts to decrease anxiety, such as addressing sleep patterns and underlying mental health issues, have also helped decrease self-injurious stims.

This last factor ties into how autism's traits interconnect. Stimming does not come out of nowhere. It is directly related to how autistic people experience the world, which has to do with their senses.

## Sensory Issues

Sensory issues are a trait experienced by most autistic people, by some estimates as high as 90%.[46] In contrast to passions, which are one of the most satisfying aspects of autistic life, these issues are sometimes considered by many autistic people to be among the most challenging.

A sensory issue is when someone's taste, smell, touch, hearing, or sight is amplified to the point where it feels more intense than would be typical. This intensity can even be distressing. What this can look like in everyday life includes wearing headphones outside because ordinary city sounds are too loud, having picky food habits because some taste too intense, feeling that certain kinds of clothing are too rough, or seeing fluorescent lights as being too bright or off-putting to the eyes.

This extra sensitivity can make it difficult to do everyday tasks. Going out to a grocery store can be too loud, never mind a movie theatre or a concert. Going to a restaurant can be difficult because they might not serve food the person likes. As an adult, this can make hanging out with friends more complicated if finding a place to eat might be more problematic. For people with particularly extreme sensory issues, this can even be heightened to the point they do not want to leave the house.

Because of how common they are across the spectrum, sensory issues hold a special importance in autism. As a 2011 review of findings in *Pediatric Research* contends, as "the neurophysiologic data mount, we suggest that differences in sensory processing may actually cause core features of autism such as language delay (auditory processing) and difficulty with reading emotion from faces (visual processing)."[47]

Although this is only a hypothesis right now, the review clarifies that the cause of this extra sensitivity is unknown. However, it suggests that the ways of dealing with them have become more sophisticated.

> Interpreting the neuroscience has been complicated by the heterogeneity of the disorder as well as the difficulty in designing tasks that can precisely probe our finely tuned and intricately connected sensory neural networks. Despite these challenges, tremendous gains have been made over the past 30 years and will guide both our understanding of the disorder as well as provide insights into how to strengthen basic processing and attention for affected individuals.[48]

Specifically, there can be an improvement for adults dealing with these issues from when they were children.[49] This can be either through repeated exposure, which helps them overcome certain sensory problems, or through adaptations that make them less of an issue, like wearing earplugs or headphones in noisy environments. For many autistic adults, however, these sensitivities persist. Some even believe it is just the adaptations that improve, not the sensory sensitivities themselves.

"When you're a baby and you're overwhelmed, you want to cry," said Mitch Helm, an autistic man in his twenties from Canada. "When you're an adult, you just avoid them."

Some autistic people experience the opposite problem of under sensitivity. They can have a *higher* tolerance for extremes of temperature and pain.[50] People around them will be worried when they leave the shower water on too hot, or they seem to be unusually resistant to a cold winter day, or they feel touch sensations at a lesser level and will stim in ways that help them feel connected to their body.

Some autistic people can manage a certain stimulus if it is predictable. For example, sometimes it's not the noise that can be a problem but how many different types of clashing noise that can bother an autistic person, like the difference between a loud concert and a loud fire alarm on top of multiple conversations.

"It's not so much the noise, it's the content," said Helm. "In a large crowd of people, I'm constantly trying to analyze everything, and that is where crowds get to me more than just having people walking by."

Sensory issues are often discussed as negative hindrances, which they frequently are. It is easy to imagine having some of the above tendencies and being unable to do some daily activities that other people do not even think about.

While they certainly can provide significant problems in a person's life, they can also present benefits. For example, hearing sensitivity can result in enhanced abilities to distinguish one pitch from another and recognize when music is off-key. Autistic people are also more likely to have perfect pitch, where they can identify the letter name of a note based on its sound alone.[51] Most people have a decent "relative pitch," which means they can relate notes' pitches to each other. For example, if someone plays a C on a keyboard, most people can match the note and approximate the major scale from there by knowing how those pitches relate to each other. Those with perfect pitch do not need this prompting. They can identify what a C is the way we know the difference between an orange and a pomegranate. This allows them to acutely detect when notes are off-key or out of tune, which can make them excellent sound engineers. Ray Richmond's son, who as mentioned earlier has an ability to hyperfocus, especially in music, is merely one such example of someone with this talent.

Increased sight sensitivity and an eye for detail can mean autistic people see what other people do not. Temple Grandin has frequently lectured about her ability to think and see visually in ways that others cannot, as mentioned in one of her most famous books, *Thinking in Pictures*. This sight sensitivity may also include an eye for patterns, a widely accepted common trait of autistic people.[52]

However, even in settings where sensory issues are a challenge rather than a gift, some businesses have started to accommodate them. It is now not uncommon to have theatres play movies with reduced lighting and sound volume. Museums, theme parks, and restaurants have also made similar kinds of accommodations.[53]

There is even a whole town called Channel-Port aux Basques, in Newfoundland and Labrador, that, before Tropical Storm Fiona hit it hard in 2022, was more famous for being called Canada's "most autism friendly town." The town, which has 5,000 people, is the headquarters of an organization called Autism Involves Me and started by converting its local hotel into an "autism-friendly place."[54] When people use this term, what they often imply is that the place minimizes sensory exposure. In this case, they modified the hotel rooms to be sound-resistant and created a sensory room where autistic people could simmer down if they felt overwhelmed. Outside the lodge, the town even has a miniature gym with staff trained in working with autistic people.

Organizations like the Autism Society of America have provided tool kits for employers who want to hire autistic people.[55] These modifications are well-received not just by autistic people but also by those who accompany them, such as parents, caregivers, and friends. In environments where autistic people are less likely to be overwhelmed, decreasing sensory input also lowers the level of stress for people who bring them to places that are less likely to aggravate them.

There are two main pieces of advice for neurotypical people regarding sensory issues:

- *For business owners, make any business as accessible to autistic people as possible. This can mean turning down light brightness or making the music quiet if not non-existent. This can mean do not have surprises, like ringing doorbells or sliding doors. At bare minimum, have times during opening hours when these kinds of measures are in place.*
- *For others who have autistic people in their lives, again, autistic adults should not be treated like children. Assume they are capable of handling something unless they show or say that they can't. If a pattern emerges with*

*them, such as a particular aversion to certain smells or sounds, keep that in mind, and do not get impatient with this. It is not the end of the world.*

This advice is a part of the social model of disability that works. The logic for businesses having these kinds of accommodations is the same as installing ramps for people with mobility issues. These ideas help to bring autistic people into society, without rejecting neurotypicals.

Not every environment can be made completely autism friendly. Being an airline mechanic will be an issue for any autistic person with sound sensitivity issues because of the inevitable noise that comes with planes. For those where no significant hardship is incurred, much can be gained by at least having times when the lights are dimmed or the music is quieter.

There can be benefits associated with sensory differences, but differences with other cognitive traits can also be turned into advantages if properly honed.

## Focus on Details: Weak Central Coherence/Monotropism

A popular theory that describes a broader way autistic people are "restricted" suggests their overall perception is "weak central coherence." Because of the perception of judgment associated with that term, some in the self-advocacy community prefer the term "monotropism," which effectively means the same thing. It refers to the ability of autistic people to focus on details but not see the broader picture — what in non-literal speak would be "not seeing the forest for the trees."

Autistic people can focus narrowly on details not just in what they are interested in but throughout their lives. A common autism questionnaire statement is asking the person to rate from one to five whether "I see patterns in everything." Neurotypicals see it as a weak central coherence when they hear an autistic person talk about minor details of a movie but miss the point of the story. Autistic people, on the other hand, consider their monotropism as noticing details that other people don't see, which can be an advantage in certain aspects of life. This may partially account for why they are more likely to be computer programmers than the general population. Both perspectives are probably correct. It is just a matter of emphasis and circumstance whether this is a good thing or not.

Todd Simkover often feels the need to tell every detail of a story. In some circumstances, such as filing a police complaint, this can be beneficial.

In social situations, however, one downside is that it can bog down the story and bore people. "One of my challenges is detail," he said. "Up until recently, I would go into a lot of detail when telling a story or explaining a concept, without realizing that much of what I said was redundant for making the desired point."

A meta-analysis from Francesca Happe and Uta Frith in 1999, two of the leading autistic researchers in the world, describes three major results from studies on this topic, all of which show some advantages, or at least preferences, to this way of thinking. It should be noted that "local bias," or "local processing" in this case, means focusing on details, which is the essence of monotropism.

> First, it may represent an outcome of superiority in local processing. Second, it may be a processing *bias*, rather than deficit. Third, weak coherence may occur alongside, rather than explain, deficits in social cognition. A review of over 50 empirical studies of coherence suggests robust findings of local bias in ASD, with mixed findings regarding weak global processing. Local bias appears not to be a mere side-effect of executive dysfunction and may be independent of theory of mind deficits.[56]

This means that autistic people are more likely than neurotypicals to have skills that enable them to correct tiny imperfections. Simon Baron-Cohen's research has shown that this hyper-attention to detail may originate in the sensory issues covered earlier, indicating that autistic traits are often interconnected and do not exist in isolation from each other. He bases this on the fact that this hyper-attention to detail is commonly found throughout all senses in autistic people: sensitive ears that pick up perfect pitch, sensitive eyes that brighten colours, and hypersensitive skin to touch and certain fabrics.

Baron-Cohen and his colleagues believe these sensitivities may predispose autistic people to exhibit unusual talents because of the level of familiarity they acquire from being susceptible to experiencing these sensations.

> Results from this and other experiments demonstrated greater sensory perception in ASC across multiple modalities. In the context of the earlier discussion of hyper-systemizing and excellent attention to detail, we surmise that

> these sensory differences in functioning may be affecting information processing at an early stage (in terms of both sensation/cognition and development) in ways that could both cause distress but also predispose to unusual talent.[57]

There is some opposition to the very idea of weak central coherence/monotropism. Even as hinted in Happe and Frith, the lack of global processing in autistic people may represent a *preference* more towards details, rather than an *inability* to look at the bigger picture. In other words, an autistic person can understand the whole point of a story, it just requires a different natural inclination and level of effort.

An experiment led by Kami Koldewyn at Bangor University supports this conclusion, showing a disinclination rather than inability to look at the whole picture.[58] This hyperfocus on details also goes beyond a broad academic discussion and into aspects of day-to-day life.

Autistic people have long been known for having issues with a trait called "executive functioning." This refers to their ability to organize their daily lives in a way that is productive for their goals and well-being. These issues may have something to do with alterations in the development of the prefrontal cortex, a part of the brain that has been linked with planning, organization, and impulse control. However, the full extent of how our executive function works is unclear.[59]

A neurotypical person might have a routine where they wake up at a certain time and plan breakfast, lunch, and dinner around their workday. They can keep a work and life schedule that keeps them in order well enough to not be swept up in chaos in the immediate term. Executive functioning also refers to the ability to regularly keep a room clean and clothes washed, among other everyday tasks.[60]

For many autistic people, this is hard.

"I have just kind of wandered off from things because of my executive functioning," said Sara Luntz, an autistic woman in the United States.

Of course, neurotypical people can be disorganized, and executive functioning issues may have causes other than autism. But on average, they have a greater ability to not let distractions impede their basic life functions.

About 80% of autistic people may have executive functioning issues, even as they can be hyperfocused in other routines that are more unconventional,[61] partly because they get so wrapped up in details. An autistic person may be so hyperfocused on making sure a certain part of their job is right that they forget about the rest of the project. It may be so mentally exhausting to remember four different deadlines that they get wrapped up in the details of one and entirely miss others.

A part of how all of this can be explained together is how many other aspects of autistic life come to make sense. In a world that is full of chaos, hyperfocusing on one thing they can manage and, therefore, control makes them feel more secure. It makes the world feel more orderly. For many people, autistic or not, having a schedule can help keep them on track, though even making a schedule can be overwhelming for an autistic person. The schedule can sometimes act more as an oppressive master than a helpful guide, which only makes them more stressed.

Dealing with order may also be a reason that breaking up tasks into small parts, whether it is in behavioural or developmental programs, has often been seen to be especially effective for autistic people. If a person can break a task down and master each section one by one, they gradually gain the skills to deal with an entire project and accomplish what they want. Particularly for autistic adults, this helps not only to keep their lives in order but also to make them happy.

## Restricted and Repetitive Speech

One of the most immediately recognizable features of autistic people to outsiders is how they speak. While they have few if any physical markers, their mode of communication after saying "hello" is often the first clue. In more obviously presenting autism, this can be non-speaking or babbling speech. In others it could be echoed phrases or completely fluent speech that merely reflects their passions and appears to be unusually unconcerned with what the other person is saying.

This could be seen as a social communication issue, as described in the last chapter. What differentiates restricted and repetitive speech from a communication issue though is its purpose. Like other restricted and repetitive behaviours, it is meant to provide comfort and meaning in a chaotic world. If they experience the world as a place to fear, many people respond by shutting down and avoiding what scares them.

There are many such verbal patterns. An early sign of autism is if a child learns and uses language through a means called echolalia. This is when someone communicates through directly parroting sentences they have heard in their environment, whether by a parent, a teacher, or someone in a movie. For example, when a child heard "Do you want a cookie" from their mother, they took that as the language necessary for asking for a cookie. They would then echo "Do you want a cookie," whenever they wanted a cookie.

In less obviously autistic people with more sophisticated language, they usually grow out of echolalia as young children. In more obviously autistic people, this tendency can last longer, even into adulthood. The repeating can remain simpler, or it can be so sophisticated that it can even make an autistic person seem like their language is more advanced than it is.[62]

One example from the clinical literature included a man named Micky who, when asked if he heard anything from his former school principal, repeated a radio interview that principal gave on autistic children.[63] He was trying to say yes but did not have the reciprocal ability to express it concisely and understandably, so he said it the way he knew how.

Echolalia can obviously be extremely confusing for people who do not understand what's going on, which can lead to them dismissing it. However, echolalia makes sense given how children learn language, which is picking it up from their environment. The difference in autistic people is how well they integrate what they hear in their environment. For kids with typical language use, they are much more able to understand the rhythm of conversation. Autistic children hear the words, understand their meaning, but have a hard time imagining how another person may hear it in conversation.

However, this is not necessarily a problem. For a long time, echolalia was seen as a defect, the sign of a damaged mind, but in the 1990s, Barry Prizant and his co-workers discovered that, in many cases, there was a functional use to echolalia that was not just mindless babbling.[64] It is an adaptation to learning language that makes sense, given that all children learn language from what they hear around them, which eventually helps them acquire the words and grammar necessary to gain functional language.

"They don't take a developmental perspective," said Prizant. "What role does this play in a person's life? What role does it play in their life over time?" The "they" he is referencing are behaviourist psychologists.

Even Ivar Lovaas, the person most attributed with applied behavioural analysis, saw echolalia as having a functional purpose.[65] In this case, the developmental psychologists were right, and it also shows how, over time, despite the many differences that still exist, behaviourist and developmental schools are learning from each other.

There are also other kinds of restricted and repetitive speech. Idiosyncratic speech is a common trait even in less obviously autistic adults. They come up with their own phrases to describe what is going on in their own heads, which to them makes sense but to others will be (understandably) confusing.

Other autistic adults may be selectively mute, have stutters, or have what is called "odd prosody," which is essentially speech that does not vary in expression or rhythm, making them seem "robotic" or socially naïve. Some of these issues also come from conditions more likely to be coexisting with autism, such as Tourette's syndrome (though the coexisting relationship with Tourette's particularly needs to be studied more).[66] This means people should be careful before saying this is autism.

For both children and adults, though it is underused in adults, these differences are often dealt with through speech and language pathologists, often shortened to SLPs.[67] These professionals, who usually have a master's degree, use various exercises to spur language development. These could include playing games, engaging in articulation exercises, and even training mouth muscles to deal with problems swallowing, eating, and drinking, though these are not usually issues in autism.[68]

These kinds of therapies are also proven to teach skills. In older children and adolescents, for example, one-on-one speech therapy showed a much-improved use of language in comparison to controls.[69] The therapy can be work, but it should also be enjoyable. "If a child is enjoying therapy," Temple Grandin said during a virtual lecture in 2021, "then it's a sign that it's good." This applies to adults too.

Beyond therapy, the speech difficulties that emerge as a way of adapting to an odd world can also tie into social difficulties with relating to other people. Echolalia or robotic speech patterns are expressions of the unconventional ways of interpreting language, themselves expressions of the chaos, which has consequences for how they are perceived socially.

For neurotypical people looking at autistic people, these speech patterns may be one of the things that gives them away as at least being different. *For anyone who notices this, they are trying to do what all humans do, just with a different kind of brain. Let them do it, do not be harsh to them.*

## Conclusion

Autism is an interconnected system, which means social communication and restricted and repetitive behaviours coexist. But they are both connected to the same thing, and for a neurotypical meeting an autistic person, this is crucial to understand.

Repetition is often a way to gain familiarity and skill. Children and adults repeat speech they hear from movies they know others have seen to bond with friends. Repetitive behaviours are a core feature of religion, like going to church or temple on a particular day, or going to the office every day and practicing a skill in the hope that one day the promotion will come. Without these behaviours, people get lost, and life becomes chaotic.

Autistic people are acting this out in a more extreme version to deal not just with their chaotic lives but with the whole world. Repetitious speech patterns and routines, interests dependent on repetition, and a practice and inclination towards small details are all aspects of autistic life that work towards this goal. That autistic people find a way to do this throughout life at all is a testament to the human spirit of adaption and overcoming the odds.

The behaviours that outsiders view as mindless repetition are often deeply pleasurable and even sensible if people understand the fundamental assumptions that underpin them. This does not mean they are always well-adapted to every situation, but that the logic behind them is as naturally human as anyone else's behaviour.

The reader should now understand something about an autistic adult's psychological makeup: what they may have experienced, how they may see the world, and how they resolve creating a world that is filled with chaos.

What comes next in part 2 are the issues in society that autistic adults must face with this psychological framework as the backdrop. Some of these are about government policy; others are about private services. Some are about employment; others are about other people's attitudes and their attitudes about themselves. Let's start with how we can make good guesses about any of these questions at all.

# PART 2

# CHAPTER 5:
# AN ISSUE OF DATA

PART I WAS ABOUT AUTISTIC ADULTS as individuals; part 2 details four major issues surrounding autistic adults living within neurotypical society.

The first issue is that there is just simply not enough known about them. Research into autistic adults is lacking, particularly in comparison to autistic children. While the amount has grown starting in the late 1990s and early 2000s, a MedLine search in February 2016 showed that only 462 out of 25,985 articles published about autism featured the word "adult" in the title.

There are different ways to measure how much literature there is about autistic adults, which can come up with different results, but the general trend is not usually doubted. Even where the research included adults, much of it is also on young adults, with older adults (around forty years old and over) being especially understudied. In this same 2016 analysis, articles about aging and autism numbered a grand total of eleven, with only four being seen as relevant for the researchers involved.[1]

Although there is increasing interest in autistic adults of all kinds, as will be examined later, far too little information is known. There are at least four major reasons for this.

- **Autism's early history**: Observations of autism in its earliest research period were focused on children because signs become more obvious in early childhood. This focus was especially true from the time of pioneering child psychologists Leo Kanner and Hans Asperger and through the first four decades of autism's research development.
- **Emphasis on early intervention**: There is strong interest from researchers in teaching young autistic children skills, which has shown promising results with helping autistic people in their lives more

broadly. Therefore, research on services has tended to veer in that direction rather than in helping adults.

- **Cause research**: There is also an interest in researching causes of autism, which — controversially — takes up a large percentage of autism funding in general. This can keep autism research away from looking into the lives of autistic adults.
- **Demographics**: A greater percentage of younger autistic people are diagnosed than older people, which makes them easier to study.

The lack of data underlies many other societal problems with autistic adults. If there is not as much known about their behaviours, challenges, and preferences, how do professionals, government workers, and autistic people decide which services work in general or for them? Or even what isn't harmful?

The harm also does not come just from what isn't known but from what people pretend to know. The lack of reliable information allows bad information to get circulated in its place, sometimes with profoundly negative consequences.

These problems would likely improve with more quality studies from academic researchers. The better the research is, the more detailed the picture of autistic adults' lives. Even the popular reporting becomes better because it will take less specialized knowledge to interpret the data.

This chapter will look at the state of the literature about autistic adults, what is known and understood, and what is important to find next.

## Defining Terms

A major problem that has plagued autism research from the beginning has been agreeing on the validity of even basic ideas about this topic, which can make it difficult to understand and define what is being studied. Even the term "autism" itself, as has been shown throughout the history of autism research, has been defined and redefined many times. Just to note its two major changes, it was first defined as a narrow Kannerian idea, and then it was defined as a wider idea of a spectrum from Judith Gould and Lorna Wing's research.

Now, many neurodiversity advocates believe autism is not a medical condition of any kind — just another kind of brain. Variations on the basic idea of neurodiversity have proved controversial, but it nevertheless shows how the concept of autism itself has changed.

The term "autism" has also referred clinically at various times to what is now called classic (Kannerian) autism, Asperger's syndrome, pervasive developmental disorder — not otherwise specified, and other names that have become more outdated. This is because researchers have discovered more about how autistic traits reveal themselves in people that the term "autistic" would not have applied to before. When more information is discovered, it changes how people think of ideas they thought they had figured out.

To this day, establishing scientifically and clinically valid frameworks and measuring them can be difficult. Of the many such ideas in autism, one widely discussed today is a concept called "masking," which refers to the theory that autistic people cover up, or "mask," their traits to better fit into neurotypical society. This could include copying neurotypical nonverbal behaviours, covering up stims, and laughing at jokes they do not fully understand.

Masking is widely reported in autistic people's own stories, which makes a lot of intuitive sense, particularly given what is known about how they are seen by other people. Accounts of masking should be respected as something that feels real to an autistic person themselves. However, as a scientific idea, not everyone in the autism research community trusts the validity of "masking," particularly the ability to measure it.

In 2020, Eric Fombonne, an autism researcher at McGill University, wrote an op-ed in the *Journal of Child Psychology and Psychiatry* that looked at what he termed "camouflaging," which is closely related to the idea of masking. While not rejecting the idea that masking exists outright, he was skeptical about "camouflage" as a valid scientific and clinical term, compared to earlier related ideas, including one grounded in the psychoanalytic tradition.

> Camouflage measures are in their infancy and still require demonstration of fundamental properties, especially of their construct validity. While research on camouflage has merit, camouflage research does not rise to a new groundbreaking area of investigation. Likewise, I remain skeptical about the claims of a vast underworld of undiagnosed, camouflaged, autistic adult females that would have been ignored. This is not to say that performing measurements with more sensitivity to sex differences in clinical

> expression would not be beneficial, but, by the same token, improving sensitivity to other differences on the autism spectrum by age, cognitive, verbal, or cultural status should be equally contemplated.[2]

When Fombonne says that camouflage requires "demonstration of fundamental properties, especially of the construct validity," he is referring to the ability to do research that teases out something called "camouflage" from other things that the tests could be measuring.

This is a significant problem for academic researchers in general. One of the most common criticisms of IQ tests, for example, is that they do not actually measure anything objective called "intelligence" but measure someone's ability to take IQ tests and are not, therefore, a meaningful test of mental capabilities.

Whether this is true or not is not the focus here. The problem this example addresses is common. In the case of "camouflage" or "masking," how does a researcher perform experiments to measure these terms? If their existence can be established, how do they know these behaviours are specifically related to autism rather than something coexisting or even something else entirely?

Again, this is not to say that masking doesn't exist. It's just currently difficult to measure in an objective scientific way, which makes it hard to assess in research about autistic people.

Fombonne's view is not the only one in the autism community. In a response to his op-ed in the same journal, eleven leading academics shared a lot of the basic research concerns. However, they also distinguished themselves by more openly embracing the idea of masking and camouflaging in general.

> Finally, the field is only just beginning to understand the impact of camouflaging on autistic people and the implications for society. We and others have shown that camouflaging is generally associated with poorer mental well-being for autistic people, *although longitudinal research is required to establish any causal relationship* [emphasis added]. Heavy use of camouflaging may have a cost for individuals' mental health and sense of self, as well as access to support, e.g., in the workplace; and may perpetuate the stigma surrounding autism.

> This raises important questions about the degree to which camouflaging should be encouraged or taught to autistic people. Fombonne highlights, as we have elsewhere, that current autism interventions (e.g., social skills training) involve teaching autistic people strategies to compensate for, or mask, their autistic characteristics. We need to consider whether such interventions may be potentially problematic for some autistic people, and there may be lessons to be learnt from autistic individuals who are resistant to societal pressure to "act neurotypical" and who therefore experience better mental health. Nonetheless, social coping strategies can be adaptive and empowering and support autistic people in leading independent and fulfilling lives.[3]

Whether it is called "camouflaging" or "empathy," "theory of mind," "functioning," "disorder," or even "autism" and "disability," debate about the validity of these terms can get quite contentious even between researchers, never mind beyond the research community. This makes the study of autism difficult to engage with, leaving a lot of open questions, which include:

- Is disability a medical or a social phenomenon? How do researchers tease out which parts of autism are most affected by biology, environment, or society?
- How do researchers distinguish between a disorder, a condition, or a trait?
- What is the goal of autism intervention? How do people define "success" when it comes to dealing with autistic people? Is it for autistic people to be more accepted in society? Is it for autistic people to learn skills to be accepted in society? Maybe a mix of both?

Although many aspects of autism are debated, some facts are seldom in dispute. The basic diagnostic criteria and the fact that autism begins at birth are two examples where there is a great deal of agreement.

One other area where there is more agreement in terms of the process of researching autistic people is the longitudinal research mentioned by the eleven academics responding to Fombonne. This is an especially important tool for finding more information about adults in general. Researchers, autistic adults, and autism organizations all agree on the potential for quality information from these kinds of studies, yet there is still a lack of them.

## Longitudinal Studies

A lot of research about autism is based on anecdotal accounts, usually stories from autistic people in clinical settings.[4] These can provide some insight into individual lives, and can certainly help in specific settings, such as medicine or therapy. However, the problem is that these accounts are highly subjective, and thus impossible to replicate in a reliable experiment. Therefore, it is very difficult to come to solid scientific conclusions from a lot of the current research on autistic people, never mind adults specifically.

In epidemiological research about autism, three notable kinds of studies can be conducted: cross-sectional, retrospective, and, most crucially, longitudinal. Because the cross-sectional and retrospective studies only look at groups of people when they are in specific moments, longitudinal studies are most frequently called for by researchers. As British psychologist Digby Tantam writes, "Epidemiologists would usually consider the longitudinal approach to be the one that leads to the most reliable results."[5]

In social sciences, longitudinal studies follow experimental variables over days, years, or decades. The goal is to show how those change and affect a group of people over time.

Longitudinal studies can take place in controlled experiments, like regularly taking blood samples to determine the impact of a pharmaceutical trial, or observations made in everyday life, like counting how many residents of an area serviced by a private water company get cancer over a ten-year period.

An example of a famous longitudinal study in another field was the British Doctors' Study by Ronald Dahl and Richard Peto, which followed the health of doctors in England who smoked cigarettes over fifty years. This study showed some of the strongest evidence that exists today of the dangers of smoking.[6]

Unfortunately, the field of autism, especially in adults, currently lacks such research. This is especially important because of the way autism affects people as they grow up. Just like neurotypical adults, it is particularly difficult to see how autism affects adults when it is not clear how it affected them as children.

Given what longitudinal studies measure and the importance of the development over time, the need for such data seems obvious. Despite this, there are problems in conducting these studies. The time commitment and resources needed by researchers are particularly difficult to attain, especially when there is so much focus on early intervention to provide treatment at as young an age as possible.[7] The research that currently exists is lacking in long-term validity.

"These studies look at a slice, a certain trajectory of individuals who were maybe diagnosed in the 1980s or 1990s," said Kevin Stoddart, a social work professional and founder of the Redpath Centre in Toronto. "It takes twenty or thirty years to have a longitudinal study. That's really the problem. In Canada, there are groups that are working independently, and we really need large, longitudinal studies."

Despite these challenges, some studies have been conducted and others are ongoing. It is generally recognized that the gold standard for this kind of research about autistic adults is based on two studies led by Traolach Burgha of the University of Leicester, beginning in 2007.[8] The first, which specifically looked at the epidemiology of autism, was published in 2011. This was later revised, and the second article was published in 2016.[9]

What was different about these studies was that Burgha's team randomly tested people aged sixteen and over for autism using an Autism Quotient questionnaire. After doing this, they went through a filtering process to determine whether those who met the criteria were autistic.

Their research goals were to determine the rate of autism among adults, to see whether it differentiated from that of children, and to create a profile of autistic adults. They found that the rate of autism in adults was about 1% across the population of England. This was not different from the rate among children, meaning the rate of autism diagnosis was likely not increasing through more autistic people in the world. It was more likely due to better recognition.

They also found that men were more likely to be diagnosed, and that autistic adults are more likely to be "socially disadvantaged," meaning having fewer social connections such as friends.[10] While there is some controversy over whether women are less likely to be autistic than men, for decades researchers have generally accepted conclusions about the rate and gender disparity in autism.

Burgha's study is unique because it was based on a random sample of thousands of people, which was specifically designed to be representative of the British population.[11] That gives these findings even more validity. Randomized experiments tend to be more conclusive than selective ones because they more broadly represent the total population.

Even though other longitudinal studies do not employ these methods, they can provide some useful information. For example, Samuel Arnold led a study, published in 2019 in Australia, that looked to measure health outcomes of autistic adults compared to non-autistic adults.[12] A cohort of autistic people aged twenty-five and over completed a questionnaire and were followed up in two-year intervals. Among the conclusions were that many were diagnosed in adulthood and that these participants self-reported higher rates of depression and anxiety. These are preliminary results as this data collection is still ongoing.

Although few other longitudinal studies have been conducted on autistic adults, the good news is that this is changing. The University of North Carolina at Chapel Hill, through its TEACCH Autism Program, is looking at long-term outcomes for 300 adults who had been in this program as children. In particular, this will have the dual aim of measuring the long-term impacts of TEACCH and examining how autistic adults do generally in later life.

> We are looking at *developmental trajectories across the lifespan and are also looking at the needs of adults with ASD* [emphasis added]. We are currently recontacting families to (1) examine employment and residential status for 30-to-60-year-old adults; (2) identify predictors of adult outcome (employment and residential status) across a 5-year time period, and to pilot a caregiver survey assessing *cognitive decline/dementia* [emphasis added] in a subset of this population to examine aging with autism. We are also studying community integration through the use of GPS trackers.[13]

Despite the benefits and increased prevalence of longitudinal studies, there are reasons why more are not being conducted. Studies about immediate gains, especially from early intervention programs, can be completed over a limited period and present results immediately. If a researcher must report outcomes at an upcoming conference, it is easier with short-term cross-sectional data gained in a matter of months.

Conclusions about how one variable, like participation in a particular therapy, can impact an entire childhood or a significant stretch of life take much longer to establish. This is not friendly to a "publish or perish" culture in academia, where continually publishing papers often keeps an academic relevant in the eyes of their peers.

To be clear, this is also not an either-or question as both short-term and long-term studies can provide good information.

There are also other issues with longitudinal studies. Tantam has written that long-term validity can come at the expense of the long-term reliability of these outcomes.[14] This relates to the issue of defining terminology that changes over time. For example, a person who is fifty years old today would be much less likely to have been given an autism diagnosis as a child than someone who is twenty today. But even if they did have a childhood diagnosis, the criteria used to diagnose the fifty-year-old would not be the same as those used now. Being autistic means something different today than it did then. Comparing results between them may not provide a constant variable over time, and therefore can compromise the quality of the study.

Nevertheless, despite the challenges carrying them out, attempts to assess autism throughout a person's life is an overriding need according to many researchers. The ability to conduct longitudinal studies over years is the only way to determine the effects of autism-related issues over a lifetime. There is a chronic shortage of this kind of research now. This trend should be reversed.

There is another positive aspect of long-term studies. They often tend to examine services and outcomes that, apart from being good for the research community, are also much more agreeable to the neurodiversity movement, as they are concerned that researching the causes is not respectful towards autistic people and focuses on fixing them rather than helping them. A focus on helping autistic people tends to bring about a better balance in research on services rather than causes, which is a deep concern in the autism community at large.

## Services vs. Causes

In all research, there is always a question of "Why should this research be done?" In autism studies, this is a particularly intense source of controversy. To answer this question, it is important to break the controversy down into two basic questions.

- What causes autism?
- What services are most effective and humane for autistic people?

This fundamental question of "why" can be broken down into two motives:

- Finding treatment at the level of early intervention (and historically, cures) and
- Assistance that can be administered at the level of local organizations, service and housing providers, and government policy.

The situation within the research world is that much of the funding allocated to studying autism looks at the genetic level — the cause question. The percentage allocated to researching services for autistic adults, defined as funding for services and lifespan research, is estimated at about 7% of total research in the United States.[15]

The autistic community generally believes that too much research is done on causes and not enough on providing services, as stated by the self-advocacy organization the Autistic Self-Advocacy Network (ASAN):

> We need more research that helps autistic people live our lives. But most autism research focuses on trying to find out what causes autism, in order to prevent or "cure" it. This is not research that autistic people want. It doesn't help autistic people that are here now. More money needs to be given to research that helps us, like research on communication, community living, education, and health care for autistic people.[16]

"Curing autism" is not the usual purpose of most organizations researching autism, even those that investigate genetic causes, such as the Autism Genome Project. That organization, run by Stephen Scherer at Toronto's Sick Kids Hospital, says its purpose is to "incorporate genetic information about autism into health-care delivery and policy development, and eventually lead to new and more accurate diagnostic tests."[17]

That being said, ASAN does have a point. There is a strong argument that a lot of autism research funding is not going into areas that could produce useful outcomes for autistic people in their day-to-day lives.

There is obvious value to many autistic adults in research on services. This could be finding out what work accommodations have the greatest cost-benefit analysis, which may help more autistic adults keep jobs. It could be concluding which therapies are most effective at helping adults deal with mental health issues. It could be determining what living arrangements are most useful, or how to fund and deliver services to autistic people more efficiently.

There are efforts to emphasize and provide these needs. An academic journal such as *Autism in Adulthood* has a view more towards these kinds of questions for autistic adults. Its articles include topics such as using non-ableist language and literature reviews about daily living habits of autistic people.[18] This journal was founded in 2019, which reflects how recently this topic, and the neurodiversity movement in general, has become more prominent. But it and similar publications are small compared to traditional research-oriented journals, the most prestigious of which is *Autism*.

It also reflects the uniqueness of this journal. Publications specifically dedicated to autistic adults in the research world are still largely non-existent apart from examples like *Autism in Adulthood*.

The quality of the research in many of the most widely read, more established journals is often high, with excellent peer review. According to the people who argue for more service research, however, they do not focus on this subject where there is more need.

This is not to advocate an elimination of cause research in general. Discovering the genetic roots of autism, for instance, has provided enormous value towards discovering what autism is and giving autistic people their identity. The research of people like Michael Rutter helped take autism from a condition caused by cold parenting by the mother to an established, mainly genetically based condition that is part of life on Earth. The concern is that the *balance* is still too tilted in favour of cause research.

Even traditional autism organizations are starting to take up this focus. One recent example was a 2017 conference Autism Canada specifically dedicated to older autistic adults, but the issues touched the lives of autistic adults in general. Many of the biggest names researching this topic came together in Vancouver. They realized that service and quality-of-life-related topics were what was most important to many autistic people, which may come as a surprise to some self-advocates, as Autism Canada is considered a mainstream group by some autistic people.

> Our think tank group will continue to advocate and support calls for ongoing funding for evidence-based research that examines autism across the life course, and with longitudinal studies that have direct application to relevant community-based programs and services for aging adults on the autism spectrum. We look forward to the continued progression of this think tank group in the use of conceptual models and robust research findings, and most importantly, the application of evidence-based programs that work to increase the well-being and quality of life for aging adults on the autism spectrum.[19]

These programs and services include mid- to late-life diagnosis, community-based supports such as good long-term care homes for elderly autistic people, as well as employment and education.

But regardless of the many debates that take place about the future for autistic people, like where genetic research could lead, what about the problems that exist in the present?

Just as happens throughout society, where information moves quickly, a lot of unsupported claims can fill the gaps for genuine lack of knowledge, whether it relates to services or causes. It is important to identify bad or incomplete information so that laypeople do not get duped and researchers do not get put off course.

## Bad Information

People dislike uncertainty. When faced with uncertainty, they often fill it up with speculation presented as fact, as well as ideology-based and magical thinking. As Kevin Stoddart explains, this tendency can also appear in autism: "You will find statistics, for example, about what percentage of autistic people are married. But we don't actually know."

In the autism world, a lot of incomplete research is presented as fact. The reason this data is incomplete is because research studies need to be replicable to test a hypothesis. A hypothesis must be backed by a collection of reliable data by multiple independent researchers, usually collected over months or years, in order for them to reach any kind of consensus.

In the absence of a lot of quality data, many half-baked statistics are presented to the public to try and give insight into the lives of autistic people. This superficially helps ease uncertainty in the short term but can ultimately lead to confusion and simplistic thinking.

Often, these are based on topics that are fashionable or have widespread public interest. They produce data such as the percentage of autistic adults who are computer programmers or what is their life expectancy. These statistics are usually not entirely made up. As covered in this book, the disproportionate computer programmer stats are backed up by studies. These claims can be based on something published.

However, the statistic can be based on taking one data point from a study and ignoring everything else in it. The full nature of the finding can be misunderstood by those reading the journal article. Even if the stat is put in context with the study, the promoters of the statistic can cherry-pick one study and ignore the general state of the literature, if that is even developed enough to determine any finding at all.

The problems can also be with the study cited. Many of them are of questionable quality, such as having a small sample size, an unrepresentative sample, or methods that cannot be replicated by other researchers.

There are many statistical claims of the kind Stoddart refers to, but even more harmful are the big-picture claims. One of the most notable examples was that, for decades leading into the new millennium, a lot of parent-led autism organizations and even politicians referred to autism as an "epidemic."[20] This is wrong. First, the term "epidemic" refers to a contagious disease, and autism is neither contagious nor a disease. Second, autism was undiscovered until psychology advanced to a certain level. It was never discovered as something novel, like SARS-CoV-2 was, for example. The choice of using the term "epidemic" was political, thought to be because the needs of autistic people and their families were ignored by the public and by governments for decades. "Epidemic" was a way of alarming people into action because it sounds scary and imminent.

This term was especially used in the 1970s and 1980s, generally to little effect. Then came the success of *Rain Man*, and the higher rate of diagnosis in the 1990s helped bring about specialized government services.

This is not a slight against these organizations, who were operating in a world unlike ours today. Many autistic people were not getting recognition, never mind support, for a condition whose full scope was not understood even by specialists. They operate in the same world as all non-profits and advocates.

Persuading people to act and donate to a charitable cause is frustrating, difficult, and time-consuming. Using a term like "epidemic" was a way they could be convincing — use the facts as they are but bend them to fit a narrative that allows more success.

For the public, it is also important to know how to differentiate activism from scholarship, and to understand both in their proper context. As a rule, there is a hierarchy for reliable information sources:

1. Meta-analyses, defined as studies that combine analysis from many journal articles on the same subject
2. Articles in reputable, peer-reviewed scientific journals (indications of which ones are best can include number of citations and can be analyzed with some training in statistics and research methods)
3. Publications from universities and other scholarly organizations, like think-tanks or government and medical research institutes
4. Reports from the popular press: books, encyclopedias, newspaper articles, public relations communication, etc.
5. Social media

This does not mean all meta-analyses are correct and all popular books have bad information. Meta-analysis can have biases in terms of which studies they include or exclude, for example. Journal articles can be based on poor-quality research while, in contrast, newspaper articles contain outstanding investigative reporting. Even in activist circles, reports by non-profits can contain much useful and accurate information.

However, when the subject is an academic topic, which includes autism research, it benefits from sources whose authors favour slow, methodical, and rigorous research methods. The closeness of the source to the original research, which favours journal articles and especially meta-analyses because it is more difficult to base findings on one bad paper, generally means that it will be less likely to produce sensational and rushed claims.

Quality academic journals are also reviewed by trained experts in the field, to whom even a good newspaper or non-profit could never have the same access. Journalists are not experts in the scientific fields they are writing about. They are supposed to be compelling to a mass readership, but this becomes a problem.

Because of its mass appeal, this way of understanding data can also lead to activism defining the terms of an academic conversation. Apart from the idea of an autism "epidemic," the field of autism has also had similarly sensational but misleading ideas such as the "autism gene" or the idea that autistic people "lack empathy."[21] As covered earlier, both ideas are based on a certain kind of truth. There is a genetic basis to autism, and autistic people can have difficulties reading other people's intentions, especially those of neurotypicals. When presented through the lens of popular media, however, they have been oversimplified and distorted.

Nevertheless, these kinds of theories can stick in people's minds, even after their social and historical context stops being relevant, as with the "autism epidemic" idea. The vaccination hypothesis, now virtually dead in academic circles, still has some following in popular circles because it gives an easy answer that fills certain emotional needs.

In order to know how to interpret research, people need to understand two simple rules:

- *If a bite-size idea seems to explain too much, it probably doesn't explain anything at all.*
- *Always have room for doubt when looking at scientific findings. For some ideas, like evolution, general relativity, and the existence of viruses and DNA, the evidence is overwhelming enough to take as fact. For most popular claims, be willing to accept debate.*

Most of these issues within autism are very complicated, with a lot of room for doubt, especially with autistic adults, where so little is truly known. This situation is even more important as it largely affects the most vulnerable autistic people.

## Older Adults

If autistic adults are an understudied group, older autistic adults, usually defined as middle-aged and older (over forty), are the least studied of them all. Francesca Happe, with other researchers, published an analysis in *Autism in Adulthood* in 2022 that shows while the amount of literature about older adults is increasing rapidly, articles about older autistic adults only account for roughly 0.4% of all sources on autism in four different academic journal databases.[22]

After Happe and her collaborators detailed the existence of the problem, Fred Volkmar in 2014 explained the main reason why there is one:

> Much more work has been done with infants and preschool children than older populations, especially older adults. This disproportionate body of work reflects an increased interest, especially over the last 15 years, in early identification and treatment with the hope of improving long-term outcome.[23]

When there is an unusually high focus on children, other people get neglected, especially those who are perceived to be "beyond help." Autistic people are sometimes reported to have a certain level of apathy because researchers and even society can view them like this.

Suz Fisher, an autistic woman in her forties from San Diego, says those in her demographic are so used to not having services that it can be difficult to imagine what can work. "I feel like if you asked a room full of autistic adults, especially in our forties or older," she said, "I think they'd say they have no idea [what services should be created]."

Research looking into the lives of older autistic adults is not just scarce but is also a tricky area of research. It involves being understanding of their general needs as older people as well as their unique requirements. It is also a technical challenge given the lack of diagnosis common in this group and the lack of reliability in trying to measure their outcomes.

Volkmar proposed one of the major reasons older adults are understudied. Scott Wright edited *Autism Spectrum Disorder in Mid and Later Life* in 2015, which may be among the most comprehensive academic examinations of this issue. In the introduction, Wright and Amy Wadsworth outline why it matters:

> While there is a substantial increase in publications related to the process of "aging out" and autism, there is a significant need to address growing old with autism, which is a missing dimension of the landscape of ASD books, publications, services, and programs. . . . "Aging out," when viewed from a gerontological perspective, is seen as just the beginning of "aging into" adulthood, and beyond into mid and later life.[24]

When Wright and Wadsworth talk about "aging out," they focus on the problems for autistic children who become adults. This is often seen as a challenge as eligibility for public services often ends in adulthood, which is the case worldwide. This means that adults are often scrounging for services, which are covered in more detail in chapter 6. Because of this unique position older adults are in, they also disproportionately suffer.

There are two major reasons for this. The first is that these adults are least likely to be diagnosed because of the lack of diagnostic criteria that existed when they were children. Therefore, they may be the least likely to know they are autistic to begin with. If they do know, they are likely to need the most help accessing services, in part because of the general issues relating to old age.

The second surrounds issues relating to older adults, including what to do when their parents have died, as they may have been the person's support structure, and there is a continuing need for care and shelter. This also includes the impacts of autism on older people's quality of, and access to, health care, as well as the common mental health challenges of aging that are especially significant for older autistic people.

Despite the overall lack of consideration, there have been some examples of attention paid to older adults in recent years. Autism Canada's earlier-mentioned 2017 conference was called Autism and Aging, and while it discussed issues relevant to adults in general, it focused on three broad issues for older people: understanding, support, and research. Its recommendations for research included some of the measures already discussed, such as more longitudinal studies and standardizing measurements so that data can be more reliable.[25]

In the meantime, other kinds of analysis at least provide some insight. Wenn Lawson published *Older Adults and Autism Spectrum Conditions* in 2015, and participated in the Autism Canada conference.[26] However, the contents of his book were telling in the sense that it is written mostly as a guide to helping older autistic adults based on experience, not research.

There have also been accounts of older autistic adults in compilations, such as *Our Autistic Lives* by Alex Ratcliffe, published in 2020, that feature stories of autistic people from age twenty to seventy and beyond.[27] Another compilation of stories by older autistic adults was released in 2021 by Wilma Wake, Eric Endlich, and Robert Lagos called *Older Autistic Adults In Their Own Words: The Lost Generation.* This book uniquely features the stories of adults roughly over the age of forty.[28]

However, the lack of research on older autistic adults and the emphasis in publishing on storytelling are still largely the case, even compared to other adults. Books that include more storytelling and practical tips can give some helpful advice to neurotypical family and friends of older autistic people. It is recommended that they seek these resources to discover how to gain insight and empathy with older autistic adults.

However, this does not give enough useful information that people can act on to help autistic adults. Moreover, the problem of a lack of research interest in older adults is really the most extreme example of what is a bigger, more comprehensive challenge with autistic people in general.

## Conclusion

Many issues surround the research and collection of useful information about autistic adults. The big take-away across ages and topics is that data is still scarce, difficult to attain in many cases, and does not produce real results until long-term studies come out showing how autism affects people over an entire life. There are passionate disagreements over the core fundamentals of what should be researched and what goals studies should try to achieve. This is not an ideal environment for any researcher.

However, as more young children are diagnosed, the gap excluding undiagnosed adults will likely shrink, as well as the ability to do proper longitudinal research with more stable diagnostic terms and labels. Hopefully, this will help correct some of these problems in the long term. Moreover, the quantity and quality of such studies with clear outcomes will also help to provide some clarity that currently doesn't exist.

Unfortunately, if the history of autism studies indicates the future, there will likely be unforeseen challenges that await future researchers. There is no telling what's yet to come, what researchers will find, and what direction it will go in.

This is also an everyday concern, however, for people who are far away from the lives of autistic people. Its impact is felt in how it is applied to services that try to help them.

# CHAPTER 6: AN ISSUE OF RESOURCES AND EMPLOYMENT

If the goal of conducting research is ultimately to make people's lives better, then it is the creation of quality resources and employment that achieves this goal.

The kinds of services that are most discussed and provided in autism circles include:

- Behavioural therapy to engage with autistic traits, whether this is behaviourist based like applied behavioural analysis or developmentally based like speech and language pathology or social skills classes
- Therapy to deal with mental health issues, such as cognitive behavioural therapy
- Disability benefits
- Housing
- Assistance from personal support workers and other outside caregivers

The creation and funding of services have historically been slow, messy, and controversial, even for children and certainly for adults. Today's service system has its roots in the aftermath of institutionalization, and while that old system has clearly been rejected, much of what replaced it is still open to question and fierce debate.

Compared to the total history of humans, the modern way of delivering these services has enjoyed only a tiny sliver of time, since about the 1980s or 1990s. There is still a lot to learn about how to do this well. Currently, many programs are prohibitively expensive, even with funding outside the pocketbooks of that person and their family. Many are also controversial in their methods, with questionable effectiveness for the goals they promote.

While some programs for autistic people show promising signs in various ways, there is a lot that needs improvement. Provisions for these programs are also sometimes clouded during discussions where some autism organizations quote the "cost" of autism because the cost of caring, educating, and providing therapy would not apply to neurotypical people.[1] This is often to the chagrin of many autistic self-advocates, who believe quoting this cost frames autistic people as being a liability. The underlying meaning, that autistic people should be respected, is deeply significant.

As a comparison, people would not hesitate to give someone with cystic fibrosis a lifesaving but expensive treatment. Why not provide the same for autistic people who need help? But showing the cost does have a constructive purpose as well. It indicates the need for services and for them to get better in terms of quality and funding. The challenges of autism should not be dismissed.

It is true that caring for an autistic person can be expensive and involve considerations that do not exist for neurotypicals. Arthur Fleischmann, the father of Carly Fleischmann, a well-known non-speaking autistic woman from Toronto, explained his family's financial situation this way in 2012:

> Anyone who deals with this knows it's financially devastating. We get some flack because we're upper-middle-class, we're incredibly lucky to have provided for Carly the things we have provided her with. I'm pushing 52, should be looking towards retirement, and I'm nowhere near ready for retirement.[2]

These high costs are often why parents of autistic children fight hard for funding and services from their schools and the government. They are needed to take care of their children, even when they become adults.

Autistic adults have even bigger problems with services than children because they often struggle to access resources that cater to them at all. Many services that should be given to them either do not exist or are not readily available and affordable. These can include satisfactory housing, which involves high costs and long waiting lists. They could also include affordable therapy, which sometimes requires intensive amounts to truly help, at costs that can be prohibitive.

After finishing school, autistic adults also have larger challenges. For instance, they are believed to be the most unemployed group of any disability category, including blind people, deaf people, and those with mobility issues.[3]

However, self-advocates, parents, bureaucrats, and researchers alike also see the potential economic benefit of autism, which directly relates to autistic adults being employed. Their abilities are becoming better understood, including their traits that allow many to excel at tasks that neurotypicals can not do as well.

The most obvious examples, in fields like computer programming and information technology, are partly due to autistic people's abilities in pattern recognition and focus. This correlation is so well-known that it has become a stereotype of autistic people, but it is also one based in reality.

There is a city in the Netherlands called Eindhoven that is known as that country's Silicon Valley. A 2012 study from the University of Cambridge noted that the population of that community had more than twice as many autistic people than at least two other Dutch cities that were not tech hubs.[4]

Beyond Eindhoven, evidence shows that a disproportionately high number of autistic people work in science, engineering, math, and technology.[5] By holding jobs in these industries, autistic people demonstrate they can use their talents and create economic value for themselves and others. Like everyone, when they have the opportunity and aptitude, much good can come.

This advantage also brings significant financial benefit to the people who have these skills. Programmers and information technology specialists make around $40,000 more than the average salary in the United States.[6] These industries contribute value to the modern world in ways that most people recognize, and yet it is strongly influenced by people often seen as burdens.

Although autistic people are more likely proportionately to have these jobs than neurotypicals, most of them are not programmers. While it is wonderful when autistic people work and contribute to the economy, they also have lives beyond that, and this is only one reason why they need services.

Some autistic people are unlikely to ever work and will need a place to live and be cared for after their parents die. The family will need extra support from society, which is especially true when they do not have enough money to take care of their child. This includes timely, safe, and adequate public housing if there is not a private option available.

For other autistic people, these services could be workplace supports where necessary. Another need is funding for technology that helps them operate in the world more easily, such as an AAC device, which they might struggle to afford on their own. AAC devices can be cheaper, but they can also cost hundreds or thousands of dollars.

Better services also include funding and access to therapy, which is disproportionately necessary for autistic people who are more likely to have PTSD, depression, anxiety, and other mental health issues. By the time autistic people become adults, they may have also internalized behavioural patterns and have other issues that may make it challenging for them to make the most of these services. However, readily available and affordable access to these services can make the difference between operating in the world with a relatively ordinary amount of difficulty or becoming an unfortunate statistic in terms of poverty, poor health outcomes, or early death. Regrettably, the status quo leads to too much of the latter.[7]

Although the need for funding and accessing these services and employment for autistic adults is significant everywhere, the situation with such resources does vary between different places. To help paint a picture of typical services, we will specifically look at the Canadian province of Ontario. Being born and largely raised there, I have some personal experience and know it best. Ontario is also picked because it is fairly similar to countries with advanced economies and touches many core issues that surround autism services everywhere.

## Ontario in the Past[8]

Before introducing specific services for autism, Ontario had a patchwork of programs for a condition that was not yet fully appreciated. Like other places, it had a system of institutionalization to deal with people we would now call neurodiverse or mentally ill. It started in 1876 with Huronia Regional Centre, the first publicly funded psychiatric institution, that eventually became a network of publicly funded establishments to house people with developmental disabilities that families would or could not take care of themselves.[9]

As covered in chapter 1, these institutions had the effect of separating autistic people from their families and reflected a time when having an autistic child held a severe stigma. After decades of decline, starting in the

1980s, the last three institutions of this kind were finally closed in 2009. They were Huronia Regional Centre in Orillia, Rideau Regional Centre in Smiths Falls, and Southwestern Regional Centre in Chatham-Kent.[10]

Before deinstitutionalization, parents of people who fit the Kannerian diagnosis of autism were often recommended to send their children to institutions. In 1974, which was the peak of institutionalization in Ontario, there were 8,000 people in sixteen institutions across the province.[11] As institutionalization faded away and diagnosis and community care became more common, public funding for community autism services started in Ontario. This period, in which the province is today, started in the late 1990s.

It started with a preschool program for autistic children with high support needs to prepare them for school. This was followed up with the Autism Intervention Program (AIP) in 1999.[12] The AIP was a broader program, but still for high-support-needs autistic children, that covered diagnostic assessments and child and family supports. The AIP also covered intensive behavioural intervention (IBI), a behaviourist-derived therapy often intended for autistic children who need moderate or high levels of support. It also covered transition supports in education, such as when a child enters a new grade or school.

Support for the AIP could be obtained either through a direct funding option (DFO), which means the government gives money to the parent for private programs, or through a direct service option (DSO), which means the government directly offered the service. This distinction has been relevant to programs in the Ontario autism funding system that came after the AIP as well.

In 2004, the School Support Program was introduced on top of the AIP to provide support for educators. This included information and training about how to make programs and resources for autistic children in general as well as create plans for individual autistic children.

From 2005 to 2015, the AIP was expanded, including support for ABA-based therapies in 2011. To put this in context, two years earlier, the federal government passed Bill C-360, mandating that ABA and IBI be covered by every provincial health plan that is funded under the Canada Health Act.[13]

In March 2016, the Ontario government announced changes to autism programs, particularly by consolidating the AIP and School Support Programs into the new Ontario Autism Program (OAP), which started in 2017. Today, the OAP is the main program providing autism services. As of late 2020, there were 45,437 children registered for the program, which includes people getting services and those on the waiting list. The Ontario government also gives the program $600 million a year, from nearly $200 billion for all budgeted government spending in the province.[14]

However, proposed reform of this system in early 2019, including an increase in funds to the OAP, created significant controversy. This is really where the source of the issue with programs begins.

The Ontario Autism Program became a system where many families were put on the waiting list. Essentially, the OAP is a giant pot of money, where the budgeted amount issued by the province is split between the children who are on the list. Between 2017 and 2019, the money went directly towards programs that would be used by families who applied for them.[15] Many families are on the OAP waiting list for funds, sometimes for years, as government funding does not cover all who apply. Around the time of the proposed changes in 2019, an estimated 23,000 children were on the waiting list.[16] Many parents were deeply dissatisfied with this system, and still are. They feel being on a waiting list wastes their child's early years, when they believe the services would be most beneficial.

The 2019 changes proposed to give everyone at least something, to reduce the wait time. The centre-right Progressive Conservative government promised to reduce this waiting list to eighteen months at a maximum,[17] through several administrative adjustments. One changed the endpoint of autism funding. Instead of giving funds to program providers, they proposed giving money directly to families, who would choose to spend it however they wanted.[18] This was administered through the Childhood Budget that offers up to $20,000 per year for children who are six years old and younger, and $5,000 a year from age seven to eighteen.[19]

The Progressive Conservative government also made the program means-tested, so maximum funding under the OAP could only go to families earning less than $55,000 per year (average household income in Ontario is $70,100 in 2020), while families would not be eligible for any funding if they made more than $250,000 per year.[20]

Public care is also delivered through professionals that work in five diagnostic hubs in Ontario, divided by geographical region. Funding was doubled to these hubs to try and shorten the waiting list for accessing these professionals. The total funding for the program was also increased to $600 million from $300 million in 2019.[21]

These changes were even more controversial, sparking large-scale protests from parents throughout the first months of 2019. Many believed this new system would deprive them of the funds required to give their children what they needed.[22] Some autism therapies, such as some ABA-based ones, would be unaffordable to many parents without outside assistance, and they believe these programs are essential to help their children. Setting the amount in the Childhood Budget to $20,000 would likely make these services unaffordable to many families.

This point encapsulates the main question at the heart of these changes. The government may have made a dent into waiting lists, but is it worthwhile if it makes access to services more unaffordable?

It also sparked further questions about the priorities of the government and even existential questions about autism in general. One of them may have been noticed by an attentive reader: *there is no mention of adults.*

## How Should Services Be Funded?

The protests got so large over the first half of 2019 that the Ontario government scrapped most of their proposed reforms by that summer. The government also took a backward step on their own goal as the waiting list for the OAP grew to over 27,600 in 2020.[23]

A more permanent set of changes has yet to come to this program. This lack of progress is still a major unsolved problem not just in Ontario, but throughout the world.[24]

The rollback of the changes has also provoked questions about the philosophy of working with autism in general, with adults as merely one part of this much larger discussion.

Autism services are complicated, both technically and philosophically, and there are no clear answers for how to provide them properly. There are two questions, however, that encapsulate a lot of what concerns people.

Let's start with the smaller one. *What is the government's role and how should autism services be distributed?*

Some people want more funding for Ontario's existing autism program, maybe with some reforms where needed, like stipulating where the money can be spent. A study done by the province's Financial Accountability Office estimated that it would cost $1.4 billion to adequately cover all of Ontario's autistic children, more than twice the current budget.[25]

This logistically simple solution doesn't demand much overhaul of the system and is especially attractive to many parents who want access to the resources they feel their children need and nothing more. However, especially during a period when Ontario is just coming out of large deficits, and in the aftermath of a global pandemic, asking the province to more than double the budget for the OAP is a hard request.

Mitch Helm, among others, said that COVID-19 made this worse for autistic people because it put the government's focus on priorities other than autism. In ordinary times, an increase to the autism budget may be an easier ask.

"It's very hard to say that autism is more important than a worldwide pandemic . . . after the pandemic I see the possibility of it becoming better," Helm said in 2021. "But unless the general public demands more politicians focus on changing autism policy and other policies that are outdated, [nothing will change]. A lot of money gets wasted through trying to make systems that will never work, work. Because we [the government] won't rewrite policy."

There are many reasons why people, like Helm, believe the existing OAP system does not work. These criticisms are not just in its current lack of resources but in its fundamental focus and structure. They believe it focuses too much on helping what they perceive as institutions that can lobby the government more effectively, rather than ordinary people truly affected by the issue. They also believe there is too much focus on early intervention and children. Anne Borden is a representative for Autistics for Autistics Ontario, one of two major self-advocacy organizations in Canada. (The other one, which Borden is not connected to, is Autistics United Canada.) She argued on the public television program *The Agenda with Steve Paikin* in 2019 that the decrease in funding for parents may open opportunities for funding outside of ABA-based therapies, which is the main type of program the money was being used for.

> We [A4A] actually formed in response to the Ontario Autism Program because we felt like it didn't conform to the needs of the community and that it bought

> into ideas about autism and autism therapy that are rather old-fashioned.... We think [these changes] can increase opportunities.[26]

While having a centralized autism program may be bureaucratically simpler than the groups of programs that existed in Ontario before 2017, this is a comparatively new and difficult change made by the government.

While the existing system may have some benefits, and change is always risky and difficult, Borden could have a point. It may not be a good idea to be too wedded to the idea that the status quo is how the government best supports autistic people. If this is broadly agreed to, there are alternatives. One is the idea of having autism services covered by the Ontario Health Insurance Plan (OHIP), which provides single-payer, universal coverage plans. This would free up autism services to be funded on an as-needed basis, like health-care costs usually are in Ontario.

The most prominent group to back a proposal like this is the social democratic New Democratic Party, the Opposition to the Progressive Conservatives as of this writing, who support a "no cap" system of funding.[27] They backed this partly because they believe that autism is a disability that should be supported along with a broader disability community. A single-payer system is a simple approach that allows for this kind of broader coverage to be more likely.

When a system exists to provide a program for one issue, what can happen is that other problems and experiences of the same person can get ignored. Most autistic people have a coexisting condition, meaning that they could have an issue with epilepsy or ADHD, and the OAP would not have services available to help with those aspects of their lives. Having autism covered by OHIP could erase these distinctions because it is administratively simple even by comparison to the Ontario Autism Program. The government pays and the network below them charges them based on what is covered.

However, there are arguments against this idea. Other disability rights activists, as was debated on the show Anne Borden appeared on, oppose this approach because they believe that autism is not a medical problem and should not be treated through a medical lens.[28] This is the core philosophical objection that leads into the much larger debate about what autism is and is not.

There is also a potentially profound policy implication. If autism is not just a psychiatric issue, more of the Ontario government would have to get involved in helping autistic people than just the health-care system. An extension of this position is that people believe other parts of the government should play a role. Their belief is that autism is an issue that cannot be delivered solely through one branch of the provincial government, which is distinct from the status quo. Currently, the OAP is managed and delivered by the Ministry of Children, Community, and Social Services, and this is largely the extent of the government's direct involvement.

Yet autism is not purely a children's issue; it also affects adults and is related to their health, education, and lifestyle, all of which the provincial government also addresses in some form or another. Moreover, housing and post-secondary educational accommodations are just two examples of concerns affecting adults more specifically.

Where does the responsibility of the government ultimately lie with autism? Whose prerogative is this? Does this even get at the larger question of what autism is? If more departments were involved, would this be too bureaucratically convoluted? Such questions need to be answered to provide an intelligent design to any program for autistic people.

There are also issues with funding. If autism becomes part of OHIP, there is much more potential for costs to rise even higher than if they are capped by set government funding in a separate program. This is true because OHIP is traditionally seen as a program that ensures the health and well-being of society, and it will be funded no matter what. This has become especially clear in a time like COVID-19.

However, areas traditionally not funded by OHIP are also crucial in this mix. Psychological services are among the least covered health programs in OHIP, including private psychotherapy.[29] This has obvious ramifications for autistic adults, who disproportionately need psychological services and are more likely to be unable to afford them.

There are calls for more government funding and control over psychological services.[30] If Ontario paid psychiatric professionals at a more competitive rate, this could shorten wait times for psychological services for people who cannot afford to access the private system. However, one argument for more government involvement is that it may also have the unintended consequence of incentivizing medical staff who work in the psychological field to take opportunities that are more competitive, including leaving for other places. Canadians are somewhat familiar with this problem as doctors went to the United States in some numbers during the early 1990s, though this trend has abated in recent years.[31]

There are also non-universal health care–oriented reforms. Many Ontarians, as well as being covered with OHIP, have supplemental health insurance[32] plans that include services like dental care and prescription drugs, which are not covered under the single-payer system. Reforms could include requiring private insurers to cover more psychological and other services related to autism.

Although this may provide easier access to psychological services for some people, there are trade-offs. It could increase premiums, which could price people out of care for other services if they then decide not to get supplemental insurance at all or get reduced coverage. This increased cost may also not be worth it to some employers who usually provide private insurance to their employees.

Given what is known about unemployment levels among autistic adults, access to private insurance may not make much of a difference in some or even many of their lives. This factor also brings up another question: If autism services should go beyond just health funding, why is there not more of an effort to help autistic adults get jobs?

Most people concerned with autistic adults would, of course, love for this to happen. As a broader philosophical point, however, those who prefer market-driven solutions emphasize that this above all else may be less costly and more effective. They particularly say this because it might decrease the cost of giving autistic adults disability services and the money needed to treat their health problems. Getting more jobs for autistic adults is also as desirable as getting jobs for others in general. As is hopefully demonstrated here, there is a lot more to consider and deal with, including the difficulty for many autistic people to get and hold jobs in the first place.

The question of how to deliver autism services is based on factors of politics and logistics, both among government and non-government institutions. It is also influenced by many outside factors, like the overall budget and broad philosophical beliefs.

The solution is not clear. There may be a mix of methods to fund and administrate parts of a system that is in many ways inadequate. Given how haphazardly this question has been addressed to this point, a better solution may arise only after a great deal of trial and error, as well as new information.

Moreover, to answer the question about economics, it is also necessary to address the second, even larger, question about providing autism services.

## A Question of Direction

The biggest question surrounding services is much less economic and much more systemic: *What is the goal of autism funding to begin with?*

The natural follow-up question is: *Which services are appropriate to fund based on the decided goal?*

Is the goal of autism funding to give children access to early help? Will this make them most likely to gain the skills necessary to deal with adult life? If the answer is yes, this is the goal that most reflects the status quo.

Therapies based on applied behavioural analysis (ABA) are the most obvious place to start when looking at this question, given how common and controversial they are. ABA is also perceived by many, especially in the autistic community, to be the most salient topic reflecting this broader philosophical issue.

As described in chapter 1, ABA is an applied philosophical system founded at UCLA in the 1960s. The person most affiliated with the therapy, Ivar Lovaas, derived the principles of ABA from B.F. Skinner, the father of a school of psychology called behaviourism, which holds that human behaviour is largely influenced by the concept of consequences.

If an action gives a person a positive reward, they are likely to do it more; if something leads to negative consequences, they are likely to avoid doing it.

What Lovaas did through ABA was apply these principles to therapy. It aims to teach autistic *and* non-autistic people skills, but ABA is particularly widely used with autistic people. ABA is often misunderstood as one kind of autism treatment. In reality, its principles form the basis for many different specific therapies. The most famous of these is called discrete trial training, where an ABA practitioner and (often) a child break down everyday tasks into "discrete" components to make it easier for the person to understand and do the overall task.[33] This could include getting a child to ask for their favourite toy that is up on a tall bookshelf, for instance, conditioning them to ask nicely rather than scream for someone to take the toy off the shelf.[34]

There are dozens of different therapies that have different specific techniques and areas of behavioural focus. These include the Early Start Denver Model (for toddlers) or Natural Environment Training (applying skills learned in discrete trial training).[35]

There is a great deal of evidence that early intervention helps autistic children retain skills that improve their lives, and ABA-based training has been at the forefront of teaching those skills. ABA providers often tout that their interventions are "evidence based," which is not wrong. Meta-analyses of ABA-based therapies generally show that they can improve intellectual abilities and communication skills.[36]

ABA's ability to teach skills to autistic children are also backed up by evidence.[37] It is also not difficult to imagine how having skills such as being able to hold more typical conversations or focus energy away from self-harm can help make life easier and more pleasant.

Nonetheless, ABA is also controversial. Mentioning it in some autistic community circles can be nearly guaranteed to start a heated argument. Its historical foundations are seen as grounds for criticism, particularly its association with Ivar Lovaas, who wrote in 1987 that autistic people were made "indistinguishable from their peers" from the therapy.[38] This goal, as one might imagine, would be a big problem for anyone who believes that autism is not something to be "fixed."

It has also been strongly criticized for its historical use of punishment as a deterrent. A common criticism of ABA even today is that it can help train autistic children to be overly compliant through conditioning obedient behaviour with threats of punishment. Autistic self-advocates sometimes even go so far as to say the way autistic people are treated in ABA is akin to abuse.[39] This is based in the fact that ABA practitioners have historically administered pain as a deterrent.[40] Some institutions, such as the Judge Rotenberg Centre, have even received calls to be shut down over using electric shocks on their students.[41] (Places like the Judge Rotenberg Centre are not the norm, but they are often shown as an example of where the most extreme application of ABA philosophy can lead.)

This is now changing. Use of such negative reinforcement has become much less common in ABA recently, and use of more "immersive" methods that get children doing everyday activities rather than sitting at a table have become more common.

"It's all based on positive reinforcement [now]," said Freya Hunter, who runs Autism Behavioural Services out of Guelph, Ontario. The centre offers ABA-based therapies. She explained:

> Behaviour is no longer bad, it's now a language. If a child is kicking me, I'm not going "He's mean, he's kicking me because he's a jerk." I'm looking at it as "What are you trying to tell me? Let me figure that out, and when I figure it out, I'll give you a functional way to tell me."

While this is true, this can come across as faint praise. Opponents of ABA often dislike the general use of aversive methods in therapy and do not approve of the punishment and reward system.

Anne Borden reflected these criticisms on *The Agenda with Steve Paikin* when talking about how Ontario's autism programs should be funded: "The way that the money was being distributed [for the Ontario Autism Program] was for very expensive and hourly intensive programs for kids, and there was a lot that was left out of the picture in doing that."[42] Among those left out of the picture are autistic adults.

Borden is not wrong about the cost or the hourly intensiveness. ABA-based therapies can involve twenty to forty hours per week and last for up to two years for a child under age six[43] and can also be expensive. In the United States, ABA was estimated to be an industry worth $1.86 billion in 2016, and annual costs of tens of thousands of dollars a year per family, per child, are not uncommon.[44]

As Borden's statement implies, whether a person is supportive of ABA or not has also become a reference point about how people view autism and autism programming in general. Supporting ABA means a person believes in teaching skills to autistic children early as the main goal in approaching autism. Supporting ABA is seen as backing the current way of funding autism. If ABA is seen as the gold standard, then governments supporting families through the high costs of ABA is the foremost goal.

This does not mean that people who support alternatives are necessarily opposed to ABA, but it can imply that they believe in goals other than those most supported in ABA-based therapies. The most popular group of non-behaviourist therapies, commonly known as developmental therapies, can also focus on teaching skills, but the philosophy surrounding that teaching is not based on punishments and rewards.

These therapies are seen as being more "developmentally" focused rather than behavioural, with a greater emphasis on how people's behaviour is a function of their development. They can include speech and language therapy, which focuses on the mechanics and psychology of speech. There is also occupational therapy, which looks at the mechanics and psychology of activities in everyday life, and social skills training, which gives people instruction and practice in talking to others. These kinds of therapies can have more of an immersive feeling. They can be done in the context of games or other activities, which can exist in an ABA-based therapy, but is not as historically rooted in this.

To examine one of these therapies, speech and language therapy, studies have shown its effectiveness in teaching speaking skills to autistic people, including one on older children. However, one meta-analysis in 2021 on autistic preschoolers said that "more research was needed" to determine their effectiveness.[45]

Speech and language therapy can also be expensive, each session costing between $100 to $150,[46] but because it is not generally recommended to be as hourly intensive as ABA, overall costs tend to be lower.

All these programs have a more interactive approach with the therapist rather than a training-based approach, which is why some people see it as a complementary or even preferable option to ABA-based therapies. Like ABA, these programs are also used with people who are not autistic and teach a variety of skills depending on which program they take.

There are also other developmentally based therapies. Musical therapy, which uses music to engage an autistic person with their environment and the people around them, is still considered an "alternative" therapy. However, it deserves mention because there is evidence backing its usefulness at improving social skills.[47] In some circles, this can also include therapies generally believed to be pseudoscience, such as facilitated communication.[48]

Although the distinction between behaviourist, developmental, and other approaches to therapy is at the core of this debate, there is also the issue of administration. At a service level, the developmental approach, if it were more widely adopted and supported by current funding, would significantly change the way that autism is funded because of its costs. If the amount of funding per child ends up being less, as was proposed by the Ontario government in 2019, it may force parents to consider options other than ABA-based therapies.

Criticism of this approach is based on scientific grounds. ABA professionals and researchers believe that ABA-based therapies are more scientifically validated, and that gearing parents and autistic people towards other methods may amount to lost time for a young autistic person's development.[49]

For adults, developmentally based help is more commonly recommended than ABA, which may influence where money goes to if the government supported autistic adults more explicitly.[50] ABA practitioners also recommend their approach for people past childhood, and some older children and adults use ABA-based therapies, but the current funding and legislative model leans towards early intervention for young children, with ABA-based therapies being the most common.[51]

If the funds were generally lowered for how much a person could get, this could promote further widespread adoption of more developmentally based therapies, which tend to be cheaper. This would particularly be the case if funding were distributed among people of all ages.

Psychotherapy is also an important service to consider if funding were to go to autistic adults. A lifetime of misunderstanding and bullying in childhood, as well as victimization and failed relationships in adulthood, can sometimes lead to PTSD, depression, and other psychological issues.

*To be clear, especially to any autistic readers, this is not a prescription for what any individual's life will be like, especially at the worst of what these conditions can present.* These problems do disproportionately impact autistic adults, however, to the point that they deserve special mention.

This means that access to therapy is critical. It is a peculiar problem because those who are most likely to really need it are also often among those who are least likely to get it. People with the most severe psychiatric conditions probably grew up in relative poverty, which statistically means they are more likely to have trauma and not gained the skills required to know what they need in the first place.[52] This is also the group of autistic people who are commonly unemployed.

Although publicly funded therapy is available in Ontario,[53] ongoing psychotherapy can often only be done privately, which can cost $125 to $175 or more for a one-hour session.[54] For many autistic adults, regular access to a therapist is completely out of the question financially. Given the potential for healing through therapy, affordable access can be highly beneficial for the long-term health of autistic adults.

But there is also another kind of service which is just as essential and thankfully, even more widely supported. Both the autistic and autism communities are in favour of increased access to diagnosis. Many people in the autistic community are in favour of diagnosis because it gives autistic people an established identity. Parents want it because it helps them know that their child's autism is "not their fault" and there are actions that can be taken to help them. Researchers like it because it gives a greater picture of who is autistic in society, which allows for better research.

This broad agreement may be why this area of autism services has been a great deal more successful than other areas of concern for autistic people. Recently, more people than ever before, including numerous autistic adults, have been diagnosed. This has also happened because of the expanding focus on mental health.

If anything, there has been skepticism of this increase in recent years, with onlookers saying that *too many* people are diagnosed. As with other childhood developmental conditions, like ADHD, there is a belief that autism can sometimes be a fad diagnosis to excuse normal, including normally naughty, childhood behaviour. However, autism has well-established and valid diagnostic criteria, so this is unlikely.[55] Even within its own assumptions, this idea is more convincing when it comes to diagnosing children rather than adults.

This is especially a problem for less obviously autistic people. For them, it is possible to get into adulthood and never be diagnosed, especially for older adults who did not have the diagnostic label available to them as children. This means that diagnosis can sometimes be missed.

There has been a large effort to have a greater number of assessment centres that screen people for autism, which can be used as a potential springboard to get a full psychiatric assessment. This need has been more met in the United Kingdom since the implementation of their national autism plan. Before its implementation, fewer than ten such organizations existed; among the first was the Lorna Wing Centre in Kent, which was founded in 1991.[56] Now, there are many more. These kinds of institutions can be useful for screening large numbers of people who may not have considered they were autistic before. Autistic adults are more likely to use these centres; children are more dependent on their parents to find out what is different about them. These centres allow people to self-direct their path.

With older adults, there is an ethical question about whether they should be diagnosed at all. For those who have lived a manageable life without a diagnosis, the question is what good this will do, and should they change their sense of self and potentially have a life-changing diagnosis when one is not needed. The consensus on this question is often that they should. The main reason is that they are not changing their sense of self; they are given a label that explains why they were who they were all along. Diagnosis does not mean a person needs services afterwards, though it gives them that option. Having an explanation for hardships in their lives may help them be less hard on themselves.

Unlike other services, which imply help is needed and therefore (usually mistakenly) a certain kind of weakness, diagnosis gives clarity. It often empowers more than it stigmatizes. John Elder Robison described his revelation of autism at age forty this way, which is not atypical for people who get an autism diagnosis later in life:

> I immediately realized he [TR Rosenburg, his friend who told him he might be autistic] was right. It [the DSM criteria] did fit me. Completely. It was like a revelation. I realized that all the psychologists and psychiatrists and mental heath workers I had been sent to as a child had completely missed what TR had seen.[57]

When looking only at services that provide direct help with the difficulties of people's skills and thinking, this diagnosis can seem overwhelming. The complexity of this problem is certainly immense.

Fortunately, there are places to start. Everyone agrees that more diagnosis within an accurate, valid framework is a good idea. Waiting lists for diagnosis should be shortened as quickly as possible.

One practical element that can alleviate the need for some of these problems and that everyone could broadly support would be finding more diverse jobs for autistic people. As is true in the general case of welfare, services provided by the government are less expensive and less needed if autistic people have the financial ability to take care of themselves.

Because many people in the autistic community are employed beneath their education levels, there is much more potential for jobs. This large and multifaceted problem can be improved simply through changed attitudes and greater recognition of autistic people by employers and society, which would establish them at a level warranted by their abilities.

Where services are provided, as will be shown in greater depth, they should also be individualized to reflect autism's diverse presentation. There should be a sufficiently broad range of services covered, whether publicly or privately.

It is also generally agreed that services for autistic adults should be more easily accessible. How this is funded, and whether through the private or public sector, is beyond the recommendations of this book.

All these imbalances between services to adults and children have profound implications for most autistic people.

## Lack of Adult Services

The Ontario government, like most others, is especially focused on children in its funding of autism services. The assumption has been that services are most effective when they are given to young children, when intervention is most effective. This also helps explain the disproportionate amount of money for children under age six in Ontario.

What this means is that public support for autistic adult services is often slim. "The adult system is one zig after another," said Steven Cohen, an autistic man in his thirties from Las Vegas.

"It is abysmal," said Kira Trinity Gray, an autistic woman in her late thirties from northern California. "When I called my regional centre, they don't even know what services there are. Essentially, the services don't exist."

Gray and Cohen's assessments are accurate for other places as well. In Ontario, although autistic adults can take advantage of some programs, the system is a patchwork, under which many of them and their families say they do not get the necessary support. This support, which can be as small as a low-tech AAC device or as substantial as residential housing, can be considerable and beyond the means of most families without help.

The Ontario Disability Support Program (ODSP) provided assistance to 14,960 autistic adults in 2019–20.[58] In 2022, it paid a maximum of $1,228 a month for single people who make $40,000 a year or less and couples who make $50,000 a year.[59] There are two kinds of ODSP: income support and employment support.[60] Income support helps people with disabilities to pay their bills, while employment support helps them to find and keep jobs.

The ODSP income support is a program of last resort; it is for people who can demonstrate that they have tried to get a job, to get help from the Workplace Safety and Insurance Board, and to get the Canadian Pension Plan Disability Benefit.[61] In other words, before getting benefits, a person must go through work-related programs. Proving that people have gone through this process can be burdensome, especially with a patchy (at best) work history that autistic adults can have. Although an autistic adult can qualify, the ODSP caters to all people with disabilities, not specifically autism. This is a problem, especially given that ODSP is *the* main program supporting many autistic adults.

"They basically design things to run programs, not to cater to specific disabilities," said Maddy Dever, an autistic person who consults with the Ontario government on the Ontario Autism Program, among other autism-related organizations. "There's a significantly high number of autistic adults who are on ODSP."

Although ODSP is the one program that offers help specifically to adults with disabilities, other programs are available that are not needs tested. The Disability Tax Credit is a Canada-wide program for those who have a disability lasting twelve months or longer. In 2020, a person under 18 could claim the credit for up to $5,003 in a year, and those over eighteen could claim the credit for up to $8,573.[62]

There are also income savings programs. For example, the Registered Disability Savings Plan helps parents save for future expenses for their disabled child.[3] Another program in Ontario, the Henson Trust, allows for money to be saved for a disabled person while not being held in their name. The advantage of the Henson Trust is that this money does not count towards a disabled person's income when considering funding from ODSP.[64]

An autistic adult can also get support through Passport, a program that gives funds to people with disabilities that allows them to "participate in the community." An example of Passport funding would be for an autistic adult requesting money for an AAC device that helps them communicate more easily.[65]

These programs can help people. However, even if an autistic adult could access all of them at once, which is unlikely, given the costs involved, the funding would likely still be inadequate to support their needs. For an autistic person who requires a personal support worker, or therapy, and particularly if they have to live away from their family, they can incur costs that are very high.

How high? The Ontario Autism Coalition has estimates for children and adults in the tens of thousands of dollars per year overall. These do factor in costs that may not apply to most adults, such as early intervention therapies, but nevertheless, costs are not trivial for many autistic people.[66] Therefore, parents of autistic adults often require outside help beyond their salaries to meet their needs.

Costs are also not the only barrier. Autistic adults frequently complain about the struggle they must go through to get these benefits. Waiting lists for these services are long for both adults and children. In an Autism Ontario survey of adults, 60% of respondents said that waiting for services was a significant barrier to getting help.[67] Social skills groups had waiting lists ranging from four to twelve months, in 45% of cases, and up to two years in 10% of cases.[68]

Housing is even more of a concern, possibly the single biggest issue for autistic adults, because of cost, necessity, and wait times. This is especially true of older adults who sometimes do not have an option to be taken care of by family after their parents die.

Passport funding in Ontario is administered through an organization called Developmental Services Ontario (DSO), which helps the government keep track of funding various programs relevant to autistic adults. Among the services DSO administers is housing.[69] Residential care homes are largely independently operated in Ontario, but their waiting lists are provincially operated through the DSO.[70]

As is commonplace, private and public supports are available, where the private options are expensive and the public ones involve the long wait times. There are around 18,000 places in publicly funded group homes in Ontario, with about 6,000 on the waiting list.[71]

Autistic people also have other housing issues. Group homes in Ontario, like in other places, can also be unpleasant, though some are well-run. This is an especially bad combination because autistic adults going into residential care are often in vulnerable positions with nowhere else to turn, such as when their families are not able to care for them.

In 2001, Kevin Donovan, a reporter from the *Toronto Star*, detailed instances of hundreds of developmentally disabled people who had experienced physical abuse in Toronto group homes and other settings, like foster care or day programs, over a period of years.

> The *Star* obtained and analyzed a sample of abuse reports filed over a three-year period. There were 274 cases in the sample of agencies, which serve about one half of the 13,000 people in group, foster or other types of homes.
>
> Based on the data, about 4% of people in these residential settings are known to have been abused in a three-year period. But there are strong indications that these reports are just the tip of the iceberg. Some cases, The *Star* found, go unreported. Staff members sometimes do not report abuse of a resident for fear of being "blackballed" by colleagues, one ministry document states.[72]

These problems with abuse in group homes more broadly remain. In 2022, a litany of issues with group homes was revealed, including kids without proper clothes and government workers referring to children as "paycheques."[73]

Regardless of the issues, there are at least places where autistic adults are cared for when their parents can no longer look after them. However, the patchwork of places currently available has not proven to be a satisfactory answer for many people. Because of the limited resources, autistic adults are often fighting for them either through long waiting lists or high costs, which in Ontario were estimated to be up to $400 a day, or $150,000 per year in 2012.[74]

Beyond issues with specific services, even qualifying for them can be a challenge. With childhood care, an autism diagnosis is often enough to be eligible for services. And yet, many children are not old enough to have developed coexisting conditions, which impact most autistic adults, including depression, anxiety, and other mental health conditions.

Developing services for adults often means addressing these problems as well. Cognitive behavioural therapy (CBT), as one example of a service, can be useful for many autistic people dealing with anxiety and depression.[75] However, CBT is still seen as a depression-related service that may not be covered by autism-related services.

Distinguishing treatment for autism and treatment for coexisting conditions can be a challenge. The major issue for the government is that they have limited resources and ultimately have to vet claims to make sure they are going to the targeted clientele.

Considering the degree of overlap with other conditions, Dever says that mental health services must be sensitive to autism: "There's only the beginning of the understanding that they're not separate things. The data is that 75% of autistic people will have mental health challenges. You see the need for mental health services to be able to support autistics."

Dever sees another reason autistic adults are (or aren't) properly served: "There's a problem that Ontario has had over the last twenty years. It's that it hasn't collected a lot of data to figure out what it needs to do to fix things. Over the last three or four years, that lack of data has proved very difficult when trying to make changes."

To get the resources, there is a need for data, coordination, and probably urgency on behalf of society and government, all of which seldom exists related to disabled people, including autistic adults.

One other way to get resources in the future may also involve more players. In Canada, this means different levels of government might have to play a role. There are some attempts to remedy this. The Canada Disability Benefit, a monthly disability benefit issued by the federal government, was proposed in legislation by the federal Liberal government in June 2022. The bill has yet to pass; though, as of this writing, it did reach the Senate. This is a long sought-after step in that direction that was asked for by many disability groups.

Over the course of more than a decade, some countries have attempted to go even further to remedy this problem.

## The Question of a National Plan

Whether the question is Alzheimer's disease,[76] women's issues,[77] or numerous other large-scale health concerns, many Western countries have implemented a strategy specifically dedicated to a particular medical cause at a national level. This is usually called a national plan. The aim of these national plans is to have the federal government fund programs and services and coordinate how a country's bureaucratic system responds to help people with these challenges.

There have been calls for autism to be included in this approach all over the world, and in some places, plans have been successfully created. The United Kingdom brought in the world's first national autism plan in 2010. It puts the responsibility for developing the plan in the hands of the

Secretary of State for Health and Social Care, a cabinet position in the U.K. parliament. The current extension of the plan, which is set for 2021 to 2026, sets out these broad goals:

- Improving understanding and acceptance of autism within society
- Improving autistic children and young people's access to education, and supporting positive transitions into adulthood
- Supporting more autistic people in employment
- Tackling health and care inequalities for autistic people
- Building the right support in the community and supporting people in inpatient care
- Improving support within the criminal and youth justice systems[78]

Scotland and Northern Ireland have since developed their own national plans, as have Spain and Malta.[79]

In Canada, there is also a strong push for a national plan. Its federal government–led consultation process that ended in early 2022 will advise the government about a potential national plan. The organization contracted to do this research is the Canadian Academy of Health Sciences (CAHS), which was founded in 2005 to conduct health-related research in general for the federal government.[80]

The three main categories that CAHS examined were social inclusion, economic inclusion, and evidence-based intervention for autistic people. Autistic people participated in the CAHS consultation for the national plan in 2021 as the consultation process was ongoing, along with family members and service providers, both public and private.

These efforts are also being promoted by advocates and have been for some time. The organization Canadian Autism Spectrum Disorder Association (CASDA) was formed in 2007 specifically to create a national autism strategy. Now called the Autism Alliance of Canada representing dozens of autism advocacy organizations, it aims to have a national autism strategy.[81] It has three autistic people on its fourteen-member board of directors, though there is a perception by self-advocacy groups like A4A that they represent more traditional autism movements.[82]

The organization produced a policy brief called "Blueprint for a National Autism Strategy" in 2019, which provides a sample strategy that includes three main components:

- Federal leadership to facilitate cooperation and coordination across the country

- Immediate federal action in areas of direct federal responsibility on:
  - Affordability and access
  - Information
  - Employment
  - Housing and
  - Research
- A cross-government approach to ASD to ensure a consistent response from all parts of government that touch the lives of people on the spectrum.[83]

In 2020, the Autism Alliance of Canada released a roadmap that talks about how a national plan can be set up and a policy compendium.[84] These were meant to complement the blueprint for what could be included in the national plan.

One aspect of Canadian politics that makes a strategy different from other countries' adopted national autism plans is that the federal government must coordinate with the provinces, which provide not only health care but also autism services.

Jonathan Lai, the executive director of the Autism Alliance of Canada, said that this fact about Canada makes developing national strategies more difficult: "It makes things slower and a little more complicated. We have thirteen governments [ten provinces and three territories], not just one." This has the potential to create a certain amount of tension as federal and provincial jurisdiction is a common source of friction that goes well beyond the autism field in Canada.

According to the Canada Health Act, the federal government can give funding to provinces for health-care expenses if the provinces abide by certain guidelines.[85] It will be a struggle, however, to decide which parts of the national plan will be coordinated by which parts of the government. Other national plans, such as one launched for Alzheimer's disease in 2019, may provide a frame of reference for how to proceed in a Canadian context. There are differences. Some of the specific goals of the plan, such as "preventing dementia," will obviously not be directly applicable to autism, as almost no one now calls for a cure for autism.[86]

Nevertheless, on a policy level, a national autism strategy would have to be more comprehensive than what the provinces provide now, and unlike current funding, would include autistic adult concerns. Lai said that many of the issues relating to adults would be part of the plan the

Autism Alliance of Canada wants: "What we really talk about at CASDA is a lifespan approach. If we look federally . . . housing is a big one, post-secondary education, employment, recreation, and society, those are the big ones . . . also taxes." It should also be noted that the Autism Alliance of Canada gives advice on policy. They do not create the rules that the federal government would implement.

The divisions among the autism and autistic communities are not lost on people campaigning for a national strategy. The Autism Alliance of Canada was formed shortly after the release of the Pay Now, Pay Later report, which was a summary of autism issues relating to testimony in the Canadian Senate in 2007. The Senate prominently featured this problem as part of their report:

> The Committee heard many different points of view on the complex issue of autism. Contrasting views were presented with respect to the definition of autism, its prevalence, the effectiveness of various autism interventions, and the need for treatment. Sometimes, divergent opinions were highlighted among autistic individuals, advocacy groups and families. This makes it very difficult to achieve consensus and to identify potential options for policy considerations. For this reason, it is clear that any set of recommendations will not please everyone.[87]

This division is also represented in attitudes towards the national autism strategy, or at least how it is conducted.

Canadian self-advocacy groups publicly opposed the 2019 Autism Alliance of Canada blueprint on the grounds that they did not consult enough autistic people and that it was "siloed" from other disability policies.[88] The self-advocacy community has historically seen people with disabilities as being part of the same community, as a group that has been "disabled" by society. Therefore, they generally see the disability community as one, and policy that affects autistic people should also be designed for disabled people in general.

Like many such disagreements, this is a matter of philosophy rather than logistics. It is not as if people disagree on the idea of federal involvement and help for autistic people, only about how to do it and under what philosophical framework, including which programs to fund and how autistic people are seen by service providers.

The efforts to make a plan are now appearing to be successful. The federal government tabled Bill S-203 in 2022, which creates a framework for a national autism strategy.[89] The bill received royal assent, meaning it became law, in March 2023.[90]

This is a statement of intent, not of a broadly agreeable national solution. Nonetheless, this is a huge step that many different people in the autism world were calling for.

Inevitably, the creators and shapers of a good national plan will be people who have influence. Historically, those who have the ear of the federal government have been more established autism organizations. Even though autistic self-advocacy groups have also gained a stronger voice in these matters, this still largely remains true.

The Senate report has acknowledged this difference of perspective, and the goal should be for the best of both communities to come into any national plan with the concerns of both reflected in the outcome. This is also just one more example of how the autism movement has almost always been divided. This next issue, however, unites everyone.

## The Marriage Question

One of the current biggest fights for disability groups concerns the perceived unequal treatment of disabled people in marriage, sometimes portrayed by them as a "marriage penalty." Under both U.S. and Canadian law, if a person is receiving disability benefits and then gets married, the recipient has their benefits scaled back or removed altogether. The assumption of this law presumes that the spouse, rather than the state, will be able to take care of the disabled person.

In the United States, two programs are affected by this: Social Security Disability Insurance (SSDI), which pays monthly support based on money the individual contributed based on previous work, and Supplemental Security Income (SSI), which gives monthly payments to disabled people based on means, in addition to SSDI.[91] In short, SSDI is like social security; SSI is welfare.

Both programs are scaled back relative to the disabled person's spouse's income when a couple gets married.[92] This also applies to ODSP benefits in Ontario if they have been married longer than three months.[93]

The criticism of this policy is the effect it has on some couples who receive these benefits. Some disabled couples do not get married because of financial constraints that come with the end of their benefits.

This fact means that it is not even effective as a cost-saving measure because the government will have to pay people anyway when they do not get married, but under a less protective support structure than they would otherwise have. This rule may be one reason that only 24% of American adults who qualify for SSI benefits are married.[94]

There is a broad scope of agreement on this issue from self-advocates to larger parent-led organizations, and signs of a growing movement to end this penalty in the United States.[95] A bipartisan bill called Marriage Access for People with Special Abilities Act was introduced in the U.S. Congress in 2019 that would end this penalty with regards to SSI benefits.[96]

Although this book has very few specific policy recommendations, the need to end this marriage penalty is one of them. It has historically been a source of maybe unintended but real discrimination and strife among people living with disabilities in general, not just autism. Hopefully, its time will soon come.

## Post-Secondary School Accommodations

Whether it is academic pressure in the classroom or the noise and disorientation of a large lecture hall and residence, autistic adults looking for extra or continuing education often wonder about the need to get accommodations to help them with school.

All autistic people face this problem, whether as children in the primary level or adults in the post-secondary level.[97]

While it is an adjustment for all young adults, autistic young adults often have unique concerns going into post-secondary school. For a group of people that has issues with variation as a common part of their condition, the change in routine that comes with going to a new place can be especially shocking, unfamiliar, and overwhelming. Even if the academics are not a problem for an autistic person, the workings of the classroom and of independent life can be a challenge to overcome.

These challenges are often thrown on top of the social issues around making friends, which are a core part of post-secondary education for most students and can often help them later in their careers.

A lot of improvements have been made for autistic people in this area. In Ontario, both the Education Act and the Ontario Human Rights Code mandate that people with disabilities must receive services that allow them equal opportunity to succeed in post-secondary education.[98]

It is now quite common for any student with a disability to have accommodations. These include extra time for exams, extensions on essays, or the option to type answers if handwriting is an issue. Another is the ability to manipulate the sensory environment to their liking, such as permission to wear headphones or use a quiet room away from other test takers. Disabled students can usually request these kinds of accommodations through their accessibility services office.

However, there are still complaints and flaws with the current system, despite the advances that have been made.

Jason Manett, an academic at the Redpath Centre who wrote his PhD thesis on autistic post-secondary students in Ontario, estimated there were 1,600 autistic students in 2017.[99] He said that this number "wasn't easy to derive," as universities there do not keep good records of how many autistic people are in their institutions. Again, another problem with data that affects services. This number is dramatically up from the 400 Manett estimated in 2009.[100]

To put this in a more recent perspective, if the number of autistic people in university was proportional to their roughly 2% share of the population, there would be around 17,800 out of roughly 890,000 students in Ontario in 2019.[101] This is not an exact measure, as autistic people are not perfectly representative of the general population. But it gives a frame of reference for how many young autistic adults struggle not just in school but in life and need better support. Of course, many autistic adults will have a difficult time with post-secondary education no matter what supports are put in place.

These numbers show that improvements can still be made. How they are implemented likely will include improving every aspect of life for autistic people before and while at university.

There are two broad aspects to university life in general: the academics, and the rest. Both are difficult for all autistic university students, but according to Manett's research, male students seem to have more problems, though the differences between males and females in general tend to be small: "Females prioritized maintaining contact with friends from before postsecondary and described higher levels of social engagement and satisfaction than males who emphasized socializing with peers from postsecondary."[102]

Manett also saw online connecting platforms as useful for autistic people: "Using the internet for email and to communicate through social networking sites is associated with higher rates of face-to-face communication and greater friendship quality. [This is] because they are used to maintain contact and arrange to get together in person with existing friends."

Manett stressed that individual attention is needed. For children, individualized education plans are a good basic, although often imperfect, model to achieve this. In university, this includes individual plans that are designed by the accessibility services department staff who take the time to get to know these autistic people.

An individualized approach reflects the diverse needs of autistic people and the lack of understanding of what generally helps them succeed in college and university.

"As for what has been successful, again, this varies widely," said Manett. "It is one of the reasons that I am drawn to one-on-one work with clients with ASD as opposed to workshops, group facilitation, seminars etc. I consider them complementary." While these other methods may have some use, this individualization approach towards autistic people makes sense. In universities and colleges especially, where one person may have academic issues while another struggles with living in residence, having a standard approach is likely to miss the mark on any individual person.

Autistic people experience the world in a more extreme way than neurotypicals, but the problems themselves are not foreign to students in general. They all require some help to deal with this new stage in their lives. Because of their developmental issues, autistic people may particularly have to work harder to develop the skills to thrive in university or living away from home. Many of them will require special attention, and if a lot of capable students are not afforded the most of life because they lack the necessary support, that would be a tragedy not just for them but also for the entire society.

*The effort to do this must be done in cooperation with each student and being attentive to their needs.* This has already been done, with noticeable progress. With more research and awareness of autistic adults, university administrators can slowly gain understanding of how autistic adults in post-secondary education learn and live.

After autistic people get through post-secondary school, then they enter another new stage of life.

## Employment

Employment is perhaps one of the most widespread and significant problems autistic people face. Given the lack of knowledge about the number of autistic people, it is impossible to have accurate figures about their levels of unemployment. However, surveys conducted around the world have suggested this could be as high as 62% to 86%, but the issues with data mean we do not know for sure.[103]

A noted problem in the academic literature from writers like Fred Volkmar and Patricia Howlin concerns underemployment, meaning that autistic people who have skills are often not employed at their level. This was a chronic difficulty for Canadian programmer Derek Seabrooke. "I took some jobs that were really below me," he said. "Including door-to-door sales, even jobs like being a clerk at a grocery store . . . those were jobs that I wasn't well-suited to so I couldn't do those sorts of jobs. I was very, very frustrated."

Autistic people face challenges in the workplace that neurotypical people do not, often precisely because of some of their autistic traits. A typical example is described in Fred Volkmar's compendium on autistic people from 2014.

> Andre is a 32-year-old man who was diagnosed with Asperger's disorder at the age of 28 years old. He was seeking therapy for long-term unemployment and underemployment. Although he had successfully completed a bachelor's degree in chemical engineering, he struggled throughout his life interacting successfully with others. In fact, his peer interaction skills were so poor that he lost numerous jobs due to a failure to "work as a team player" or "get along with co-workers." Co-workers reported that Andre was rude, abrupt, disorganized, and frequently came to work disheveled without having showered or even brushed his teeth. His personality and lack of personal hygiene skills made others at work avoid him.[104]

Some autistic people have fundamental challenges that will likely make finding a job a challenge throughout their lives; others can overcome their differences, especially with support. These can arise before the autistic person ever gets the job, for example, with executive function issues needed to look for work. The lack of connections an autistic person may have or be comfortable using can be a significant barrier as many jobs are discovered this way. Even when an autistic person gets something of a break, a job interview can be notoriously difficult territory for them to navigate.

These kinds of skills, which have nothing to do with their capability to do a job, can be a real problem, even for autistic adults who have learned a decent number of social skills. Some issues with these competencies can be innate, others can be caused by trauma.

"When I was younger, I had frequent meltdowns, mostly because of bullying or too many demands being placed on me," said Michelle Harris, an autistic woman from Texas in her early thirties. "I have always had a tendency to overshare my past, as well as to 'infodump' on people regarding my special interests. My social skills have improved, but not enough to do well in job interviews."

Job interviews are littered with all kinds of potential problems for many autistic people. These arenas tend to heavily favour those with conventional social skills, such as looking people in the eye, speaking confidently, and shaking hands (at least before COVID-19 and virtual interviews becoming more common).

Worrying about whether an autistic adult is a good fit for an organization can sometimes keep them from being hired in the first place. Saying the wrong thing or volunteering too much information in a job interview, which is disproportionately a risk for an autistic person, can get them in trouble. Their personality and idiosyncratic way of looking at the world can also lead them to give answers to questions that make complete sense to them but are alien to the interviewer. This inability to "translate" what they are thinking, or even to get confused and garbled, can lead to problems when convincing an employer that they are right for a job.

Other problems for autistic adults arise once they have a job. Many require accommodations to address specific issues. These can be sensory related or to do with interruptions, as they have trouble changing focus on tasks when a need might arise or dealing with people. If these problems are minimized, autistic people can be excellent employees in that field.

Most workplace accommodations for all disabilities are relatively cheap, with the majority costing under $500 as a one-time expense, according to

Canadian estimates.[105] For many employers, this is relative pocket change. These can include text-to-speech software, a private place for people to work away from noise, or even just a pair of earplugs. Despite this relative ease of cost and access most of the time, many autistic people find it difficult to gain the confidence to ask for such help. Regardless of the requirements under legislation like the Accessibility for Ontarians with Disabilities Act, which many Ontario workplaces must comply with by 2025, getting these accommodations in practice can be difficult.[106]

Without these accommodations, autistic people can find it challenging to regulate their sensory issues and emotions at work. All employees must do this, of course, but autistic people have much greater potential for such issues because of their level of sensitivity.

There are also issues with workplace social culture. Depending on how much an autistic person specifically struggles with social skills, they may be more likely to be isolated from other people. They may also turn off co-workers by being socially naïve, having different interests, or lacking social experience that most adults have already had due to developmental differences. Whether these co-workers are also misunderstood, which is at least partly possible, does not lessen this challenge for autistic employees.

In a modern service economy, autistic teenagers and young adults can be at a significant disadvantage because their front-facing service positions are often an entry point into the job market. They are demanding on the weak points of autistic people, such as talking with others, regulating emotions, and dealing with rapid change.

Not all jobs are like this, and some autistic young people may be lucky enough to get ones that play to their strengths, although their areas of weakness can still pose challenges in many workplaces. As difficult as solving this problem can be, reshaping the economy is even more challenging. If an autistic employee gets a front-facing service job, there are ways to make that more tolerable, such as being particularly explicit and taking extra time with instructions and offering more opportunities for breaks.

*Employers should be aware of the strengths of autistic employees that make some adjustments worth it for them.* These can include many positive traits, such as honesty, tending to be punctual, not participating in workplace gossip and drama, and following instructions (if the instructions are made clear to them).[107] If autistic people sometimes say the wrong thing to someone, they seldom truly mean to do harm.

Although all employees have potential struggles and a learning curve, autistic employees can have different and more glaring issues for an employer, but fundamentally they are not different. Like everyone else, if autistic people are given time to grow, they can be great employees in just about any field.

Therefore, it is so important to think of ways they can thrive in the workplace, at all levels from entry-level up the chain of command.

## Ways to Help with Services and Employment

This book does not make many definitive claims about how to fix service systems for autistic people. It is much more intent on getting people to think about these highly complex issues rather than impose answers.

Any recommendations from a single source are likely to be missing important details. However, some intelligent choices and goals could be undertaken that, if achieved, would make a significant difference. These include:

- Giving autistic employees and students more patience and direct feedback regarding their growth — the long-term benefits may be significant
- Focus on making living accommodations safe and expanding their numbers
- Giving more options, such as the option for video lectures to avoid large gatherings, which allow autistic people to learn in environments that fit their needs

Beyond specific solutions, it is especially salient to address how the research community, the service sector, and autistic people are currently talking about solutions and what their difficulties are in coming to a consensus.

Whether it is at the government or private sector level, the two basic questions related to these issues are what kinds of services are the most successful, and what are the best ways to fund them. The services that can be effective are very diverse, just like the community itself. One aspect of successful services is that they get autistic people involved in the community. It is not uncommon for autistic adults to have solitary, sedentary lives, which, for anyone, is likely to reduce physical and mental health.

Many autism organizations provide group activities specifically to serve autistic adults. The Geneva Centre for Autism in Ontario, a traditional autism agency, and Autistics United Canada, an autistic-led organization, both provide regular game nights, social events, and activities like swimming or music.[108] These can even be groups not specifically for autistic people, but regular activities that appeal to an autistic adult's interest and also give them a sustained and reliable sense of community.

"I think the types of services that are best are the types of services that help to develop communities of support," said Barry Prizant, talking specifically about two autistic theatre companies out of Los Angeles and Providence, Rhode Island, that he is involved in. These are meant as ways to give connection and an activity for autistic adults.

With regards to employment, Prizant, like many others, also is stringent about helping autistic people find what they're good at even before they become adults. This can give them clarity and focus so they can use their skills to support themselves. "Any human being has a better quality of life if what they do is a good match for their brain structure," said Prizant.

There are more broad, relatively radical solutions. Many autistic self-advocates support the idea of universal basic income.[109] Because of the number of autistic people who may have to live on disability benefits and are unable to work, having a guaranteed payment that is not justified by proving one's disability status is seen as attractive. These people would receive a form of support that they do not have to justify through difficult and frustrating issues with bureaucracy, such as proving their disability.

At a certain level, and without the stigma of welfare that only some "dependent" people receive, autistic people's basic quality of life may improve to where they can build themselves up. This may also be an ancillary benefit for a policy discussion that has much broader implications, and therefore could attract more political buy-in. If the entire society can benefit, the politics become more straightforward than if the discussion is just about autism or even disability.

Finally, whatever the whole society decides to do, because this is ultimately a societal issue, it will likely not go anywhere without the buy-in of autistic adults themselves. Autistic adults are still adults. They need to be assumed to be competent before it's evident they are not. While they may need more support than many neurotypicals, if they are not feeling good or supported by the services around them, any other services or support that are offered will not be productive.

## Conclusion

Many autistic adults, their parents, and professionals who represent them all agree that the system around autism has significant flaws, in Ontario and likely elsewhere. Many people believe the current system focuses more on trying to change autistic people rather than helping them navigate a world they inevitably will have to face. There is a point to be made about emphasizing early intervention, but the system does not provide sufficient focus on a broad enough group of people.

Most autistic people are adults, and this group is not given enough attention by the research community and service providers. Many of them need help with considerable challenges and expenses, and they need it as soon as feasible.

How should this be done? It is difficult to say. Governments have limited budgets, and the private sector has its own challenges in providing affordable services at a low cost, including scarcity of workers and demands on their time and skills that require payment from somewhere. There are likely some solutions out there, but they will involve a lot of work not just to implement but to even conceive.

It's also particularly difficult to answer this question when everyone has a different philosophy about what the goals are. Is it to teach autistic people to "function" in society as early as possible? Or is it to help society understand and treat them in ways that are not too stressful? There are important groups of people who have diametrically opposed views on this subject.

There is also a problem of organizing that hurts autistic people, including adults. This is a large population of people, many of whom desperately need help, but they lack the effective organizational capacity to push for services at this point. In some cases, they do not have the capability to advocate for themselves because of challenges in their own lives. They need better representation, which probably includes help from non-autistic adults. The need for co-operation is clear. Only then can there be an effective push for services that are really needed.

This task is much more difficult than it sounds because of the divisions between traditional and self-advocacy groups. A unified effort from everyone who has a stake in the issue will be a much more effective lobbying effort than one that is divided and will give parent-led groups an advantage because they have more money and more lobbying power. These parents deserve a voice, but so do autistic people themselves.

A new national plan with federal government coordination may provide help to autistic people, if not also to adults. There is a lot of promise. However, any plan will likely alienate one side or another, which means that the CAHS recommendations and the ultimate by-product of them will have to be deeply considered. Without at least a broad agreement that everyone can live with, the plan will not happen as anyone would hope.

For many autistic adults, their priorities feel low down on the list to other people in society. While there has been great improvement in this field, especially for children, the focus on early intervention has left behind many people who need help. There is a lack of purpose and scope in the provision of autism services that particularly affects adults.

To bring about this change, the entire society, from strangers to immediate family, needs to not just be aware of this subject but also accept autistic people.

## CHAPTER 7:
## AN ISSUE OF PUBLIC UNDERSTANDING

RESEARCH AND SERVICES RELATED TO AUTISM are most helpful when the rest of society is aware of them and what they are used for. The better educated that people are on who autistic people are and what their issues are, the more likely they are to interact and help in ways that more often fit for them. Family will be able to understand what an autistic member needs, the public will be able to understand a meltdown and how to treat it, and service providers will know how to deal with autistic people and find help that works well.

While public awareness of autism has increased over the years, and this has helped autistic people a great deal, many still find issues with ignorance and mistreatment to varying extents. This can be as commonplace as a first date with someone who becomes turned off after they say something a little too honest. At its worst, it can even involve an abusive family member who never bothers to learn about autism and makes every day a nightmare for the autistic person.

Situations like these most extreme, even criminal examples are usually made worse by the autistic person's issues with communicating with others, which is necessary to tell someone about your problems or to report them to the police, to tell a teacher what they need if they're a student, or to tell a family member how to help them when they're in distress.

Sometimes, it can even be medical practitioners who do not understand autism enough to help their autistic patients. Of course, they almost always know that autism exists, but they do not understand it at an adequate level, which significantly impacts the lives of autistic people who interact with them.

This is being addressed among activists. The issue of public awareness is a common one within many medical condition–related charities, and always has been. In big non-profit organizations, whole departments are dedicated to social media, media relations, and other awareness initiatives.

What's different now is that these organizations, including autism-related ones, have started to have higher standards. In recent years, autistic people have gone away from the idea of awareness to the idea of acceptance. April, which has historically been called "Autism Awareness Month," has been increasingly called "Autism Acceptance Month" by both autistic and autism charities.[1] The underlying idea is that the public needs to go beyond just knowing that autism exists and start accepting autistic people for who they are and integrating them into society.

When it comes to "public understanding," this can mean different things at different levels of society, whether it is family, friends, employers, or strangers who reflect an entire culture.

So, who needs to understand what?

## General Public

At the broadest possible level, which is the way autistic people are treated by the public, there is some evidence public perception is improving all over the world. A study carried out in Saudi Arabia in 2015 showed that 88% of its population had heard of autism.[2] In Australia, a 2019 survey of 1,054 people showed that an overwhelmingly high percentage (more than 80%) of people not just knew about autism but had a relatively advanced knowledge of it. This knowledge, crucially, may also reflect that they had a positive attitude towards it.[3]

Surveys are often seen as an imperfect form of data collection, full of potential issues with sample sizes and truly randomized sampling. Political polling, to take a common example, is still critiqued for this reason.[4] But enough polling can show clear trends over time, and the trends of these surveys show some clear developments: most people are now at least aware of the existence of a condition called autism and some of its aspects.

While it is great to know about autism, and even in some places to have positive feelings about it, acceptance and respect are a whole necessary step that has not developed as much. How autism is viewed, at least according to polling, differs from place to place. In some, positive attitudes towards it and even knowledge in general can be sadly lacking. A study comparing China and the United States, for instance, indicated that knowledge of autism was much higher in the U.S., showing 91% of Americans had "adequate" knowledge of autism compared to 61% of people in China. Even more importantly, many more people held views the author deemed stigmatizing towards autistic people in China, about 38%, compared to about 14% in the United States.[5]

In other countries, these negative views of autistic people get even darker. A study in Taiwan, for example, indicated more than half of mothers would abort their children if they discovered pre-birth that their child was autistic.[6] This reflects the "autism is a burden" attitude that was much more common before advances were made in clinical understanding.

This trend holds up elsewhere as well. In the Saudi Arabian study that found most were aware of autism, 41% of respondents said their knowledge of it was "weak."[7] One study of pediatricians in Iran showed that they had better knowledge about autism than the general population, but there were still problems with understanding autism even among this group.[8]

In Western countries, there is also the movement to not have autistic adults even viewed legally as adults, which is a long-standing fight that does not seem to be letting up. The autistic community in Canada has fought against proposed changes such as one that defines "children" as including disabled adults in line with the definition of "child" under the Divorce Act. This was introduced in Ontario in 2021.[9]

This development says a lot about how autistic adults can be viewed even in the modern day. They can be viewed as people who don't just have challenges, like any person with a disability, but are incapable of making decisions for themselves. Many people with disabilities do warrant lifelong care by others, although a caregiver will have to make decisions for them in at least some cases. A major criticism of this proposed change is that these situations are already covered in Ontario through the 1992 Substitute Decisions Act, which defines a person who is "unable to manage property" for instance, this way:

> A person is incapable of managing property if the person is not able to understand information that is relevant to making a decision in the management of his or her property, or is not able to appreciate the reasonably foreseeable consequences of a decision or lack of decision.[10]

This definition is not as stigmatizing as labelling them as children and does consider individual circumstances. This standard allows much more autonomy for autistic adults.

While many Ontarians are not even aware of this act, as it doesn't directly affect enough people to become a front-page political issue, the perception of autistic people implied in this development could be significantly impacted by the government carelessly defining a dependent in this way. More people should be aware of the capabilities as well as the challenges of autistic people because these arise even in high-level government discussions and policy, never mind just in public life.

While the numbers may differ by location, autistic people everywhere complain about their doctors' lack of real understanding about their condition. These professionals should know more about autism to inform their practice, given its prevalence.

This gap in true understanding underpins the change in how both autism and autistic organizations campaign. Organizations such as the Autism Society of America in the autism community and ASAN in the autistic community are going from awareness to acceptance, which reflects what they now see as the greater priority in public understanding. Their message is that neurotypical people should treat autistic people as if they're no different in any fundamental way from them. This is a message most people would accept in principle, but in practice it is often much more complicated.

Based on these studies, discrimination against autistic people is not due to conscious dislike of a particular group. Many neurotypicals do not know or think enough about autistic people to be consciously bigoted against them.

Especially in cases where autism's presentation is less obvious, their identity is not always readily evident in their appearance. It is only after getting some superficial initial impressions, or even in some cases behaviours that can only be detected after repeated encounters, where they make judgments.

The ways autistic people can reveal being different — like stimming, certain kinds of body language, or speech patterns — are often perceived by neurotypicals as "weird," "unpredictable," or "eccentric."

This has real-world impacts. Impatience and prejudice from the public can make renting an apartment, ordering a meal, and meeting new people difficult and uncomfortable. Even the United Nations has recognized this trend around the world.[11] For certain people, specific tasks can be nearly impossible, and some of these issues have at least as much to do with the other person's attitude as it does with the autistic person.

Deb Wrightson sees these misunderstandings as a pervasive problem:

> I think autism is massively misunderstood, and people don't think I look or sound autistic. I'm too clever to be autistic, I make eye contact, I smile at people. Very few people have heard of masking, which has been something I've done all my life (without knowing I was doing it). Teachers definitely don't understand autism. They're nowhere near enough educated on it, which makes it extremely traumatic for autistic kids in school.

These stigmatized traits can also present themselves when someone is desperately trying to fit in, which makes an autistic person feel the rejection even more. All humans perceive difference, and autistic people are not incapable of prejudice themselves. But they also experience it more than most people.

These perceptions from neurotypical people have also received some academic attention. Noah Sasson, previously mentioned for his work on the double empathy problem, led a study about neurotypicals' attitudes towards autistic people. His team found that they were turned off by autistic people, usually by split-second decisions — with one situational exception.

> Here, across three studies, we find that first impressions of individuals with ASD made from thin slices of real-world social behavior by typically-developing observers are not only far less favorable across a range of trait judgments compared to controls, but also are associated with reduced intentions to pursue social interaction. These patterns are remarkably robust, occur within seconds, do not change with increased exposure, and persist across both child and adult age groups. *However, these biases disappear when impressions are based on conversational content lacking audiovisual cues, suggesting that style, not substance, drives negative impressions of ASD* [emphasis added].[12]

In other words, the off-putting feature of autistic people is not the content of their speech; it is the way they appear. There is an immediate repulsion to perceived difference, because along with unfamiliarity, it can mean threat. On the telephone, where judgments about eye contact are not possible, people will not feel that way.

It is a common trait of humans to notice difference.[13] This is possibly even useful in some ways, and therefore it is understandable and not necessarily worthy of harsh judgment. But human nature does not always create ideal outcomes, especially for people who have non-threatening differences like autistic people.

Given the realities of where people are at with prejudice and how deeply rooted it is, what can be done to improve public perception?

If there is one major change that *has* altered how the public perceives autism, it is likely the rate of diagnosis. Neurotypicals are now much more likely to know someone who is autistic. There are also more autistic people who can vocalize their own condition, given the profile of autistic people and their awareness of who they are.

One 2020 study indicated that increased familiarity improved relationships with autistic people in the United States.[14] While this appears initially to contradict Sasson's findings, as he says more exposure does not necessarily improve perception, this increase in diagnosis means that autism inevitably touches someone's life. This factor makes a big difference.

It is easier to accept autism when a person's friend, brother, or co-worker is known to be autistic. When the autistic person is a stranger, they're different and dismissible; when it is someone known, they're familiar and it would be cruel to dismiss them. This fact forces a person to confront their own prejudices because rejection stops being easy.

A familiar historical parallel to many readers is when gay people started to come out in greater numbers, as the familiarity they gained in people's ordinary lives led the way for the dropping of prohibitions on gay people to get married, join the military, and be recognized under human rights protection laws.

Although this process started long ago for autistic people, there are many more avenues for increased understanding among neurotypicals. The first is that autistic adults are often given much less sympathy than children. More is known, both by researchers and the public, about children, which helps perception.

However, autism is a developmental condition, which in lay terms can sometimes seem to be what is called "immaturity." Children are expected to be immature; adults are not. When an autistic or neurotypical child makes a social mistake, it is treated with more leniency because of their age. Adults are thought to already understand social rules that children have yet to learn.

If it is only the outside presentation that people notice, they are less likely to think about autism when they catch a social mistake or see a person get visibly bothered by something. That person's attempts to explain can also sometimes be seen by others as "making excuses." It can be difficult for a non-autistic person unfamiliar with how autistic adults present to make that leap. Autism is lifelong, however, and there will always be difficulties and differences in autistic people, regardless of age, that neurotypicals may not understand. Therefore, more diagnosis and education are necessary.

This attitude, which has a certain neurodiversity perspective, is also sometimes correlated with other attitudes, including one that has historically been popular: to try and help autistic people seem more neurotypical. This can be through classes, training, and, in the case of many adults, osmosis, to help them emulate neurotypicals in their behaviours to seem less different and make it more likely they will be treated better.

The biggest problem with this idea is that it is extremely offensive to the autistic community, which frequently emphasizes autistic people being able to be themselves above almost everything else. It's not autistic people who should change, they say, it's society's attitudes towards them.

The fear from the autistic community is that an autistic person can become overly compliant and hide who they are, which causes psychological problems of its own. Although this is true to a large extent, at its extremes, it is also absolutist. In such a complicated condition like autism, it is impossible for a stranger to really understand everything about an autistic person, especially one with subtle presentation.

There is a way to compromise. Broader understanding can improve the lives of both autistic and neurotypical people who cross paths. In an imperfect world, however, it makes sense to give autistic people at least some skills that help them cope with the neurotypical world as best as they can. This is not expecting autistic people to be neurotypicals or to pretend to socialize like them. The goal is to do the maximum that is necessary to help autistic people do what *they* wish to achieve.

Whatever the methods chosen, which have largely been a mix of accommodation and assimilation in the last thirty years, the arc of history has gone in the right direction. As autistic people form distinct groups while still being connected to society, and as more people are diagnosed, the ability for the rest of society to understand and accept them grows. The ability to provide services that respect autistic people and help them cope also grows.

This broader perception is also dependent on how autistic people can manage their lives at more local levels.

## Jobs

Apart from the concerns about unemployment, legal, and accommodation, the perception of bosses and co-workers is a still pressing among autistic adults. Even for credentialed adults, the evidence suggests that there are significant barriers to the work world from attitudes towards autistic people.[15]

A study reported in the *Scandinavian Journal of Disability Research* by Jonathan Vincent, a senior lecturer at York St John University, looked at this question and found this about employer attitudes towards autistic people:

> Employment immobilities were further exacerbated by experiences of employer discrimination towards autistic graduates throughout recruitment processes alongside non-human "actants," such as job adverts, application forms, and interviews that create obstacles for autistic applicants. . . . These findings are significant given the increasing number of autistic young people entering the higher education system around the world and the wider evidence that suggests mal-employment or unemployment for this population.

It should be noted that this study had a relatively small sample size of autistic students, with only twenty-one interviewed. Vincent himself also says that "there is still much work to do to develop more theoretical applications," so this should not be taken definitively.[16] At least from the reports of autistic adults, they are familiar with the content of Vincent's findings, either among the people they know or within their own experience.

M., the woman in her mid-forties from Canada mentioned earlier, has three university degrees and now works as a computer programmer after having many other jobs, including being a bus driver. She said that, despite her technical knowledge, she has faced issues in the workplace from employers because of autism. One instance, where a vacancy occurred at a church where she had volunteered as a musician, was so impactful that it sparked her to get her diagnosis.

A person who left a paid position at M.'s church "assumed she could leave easily because I was there and could just take over," M. said.

> The pastor likewise said the same thing. But the hiring committee said they wouldn't hire me, and they gave me a whole bunch of reasons, which to me were not reasons at all. Stuff about things I should have known I was supposed to do but I didn't do. They said I lacked initiative. But the thing is, I didn't not do it because I lacked initiative, I didn't do it because I genuinely didn't know.

A story like this is painfully relatable to many autistic people. When these traits are the difference between making a living and not, it can create stress, dependency, and even feeling like a failure. In undiagnosed autistic people, like M. at the time, this is based on something that is not known to the person, which only increases the frustration.

Sometimes this fear of discrimination is why autistic people do not disclose their autism to employers. Whether they should make such disclosures is commonly debated in autistic circles.[17] In an ideal world, this question wouldn't need to be asked, as autistic people would be able to talk about autism like they go to the movies. In the world today, the most common answer is "it depends."

It will depend on the type of employer a person is applying to work for, as some industries are more accommodating to an autism diagnosis than others. It will depend on whether the person will need accommodations to do their job well. It can even depend on how people socialize in that workplace. Are other co-workers likely to look down on an autistic co-worker for potentially receiving "special treatment" or see autism as an excuse? All of this can impact how open an autistic person should be, or even can be.

It is illegal to discriminate based on disability under Section 15 of the Charter of Rights and Freedoms in Canada, and laws like this exist in other industrialized countries, even if they are not entrenched in the constitution.[18] At least at anecdotal levels, autistic people still widely report issues with the attitudes of people in their jobs.[19] Many of these issues are probably not related to conscious discrimination but with attitudes towards difference. There can be the attitude, whether before or after an autistic person is hired, of "Can I work and get along with this person?" which can often mean in practice that autistic traits are excluded from those criteria.

It is considered unreasonable to discriminate because of a protected category, like disability, but it is considered reasonable to discriminate because they are not a "good fit." In practice, not being a "good fit" in the workplace can be reflected in autistic people having difficulties in making small talk or demanding a little bit more of a manager's time because they must clarify and ask more questions, as autistic people might be more prone to do. It's not overt discrimination, but these workplace issues are related to their autism.

One anecdotal case is reported in an article for the London School of Economics. Brett Heasman talks about how the double empathy problem is an issue for autistic employers. The employers that he talked to were not ill-intended, but it was also clear that they were not understanding enough of their autistic employees to really allow them to do well in their workplaces.

> From the employer's perspective, they were very keen to show that they had been adapting to his particular way of working within what they perceived to be reasonable adjustments. However, there were still some points that I had to clarify to the employers which highlight the "double empathy problem" in action.
>
> For example, it emerged that in meetings, the autistic employee would often misunderstand what had been said. In response, the employer stressed that they had no problem with the meeting being stopped if the autistic employee wanted to ask a question or clarify a point of discussion. Yet this is a problematic assumption, because the autistic employee may not realise a misunderstanding has taken place until much later, when it had manifested into a problem, and even if he did recognise in the moment

> that there was a misunderstanding, it should not be assumed that he would be able to "speak up" instantly.[20]

Heasman goes on to say that speaking up can be an especially difficult skill for an autistic person as it involves social skills that can be complicated for them, such as timing and leaving in only relevant details. Of course, this can be true, but an employer's response could be that the autistic person themselves must clarify and explain, to the best of their ability, what they do not understand, whether it is in or outside of the meeting. An employer cannot read someone's mind, and therefore, they cannot know every possible instance where a misunderstanding could happen.

This is where relationships at work between autistic and non-autistic people can get difficult. Unless a neurotypical knows how to get inside an autistic person's head and vice versa, which can take a lot of work and curiosity, it can sometimes be seen as more hassle than necessary to work between the two. This isn't good enough, of course. As autistic people tend to be the ones who suffer most from these imbalances, it is worthwhile for neurotypicals to try and understand a person who could end up being a valuable employee.

There is also the other question of how an autistic person receives feedback. As Heasman notes, an autistic person is more likely to be dealing with low self-esteem because of the issues with criticism and abuse they're more likely to have had in their life. This can make even well-meaning criticism sting more.

> Another challenge was the employer was very focused on developing strategies for the employee to embrace and work with "constructive criticism" in order to improve the way in which the team worked as a whole. I suggested that it might also be a good idea to run over the positive things which the autistic employee had done. From the employer's perspective, this had not seemed particularly necessary because many of the positive aspects were deemed obvious. However, when I spoke to the autistic employee, it was very clear that he had no idea what it was that he did well, and because of his low self-esteem, would often downplay compliments.[21]

*This should always be kept in mind by a superior at work.* Likewise, for autistic people, who can be overly honest, learning to couch criticism in a way that does not make people feel bad is also a useful skill.

After all, Heasman and others are writing based on a *double* empathy problem, which means understanding communication can go both ways. This is whether an autistic person is an employee, which is often assumed in discussions about autism and employment because this is more common, or whether the autistic person is themselves a superior, where having good people skills is especially valued.

Thankfully, there are programs available to address such issues. One newer one, AUsome Training, offers online seminars given by autistic people for parents, teachers, and professionals. Their training is precisely on how to have good relationships with autistic people.[22]

AUsome's view is plainly one based on a neurodiversity framework, and the presentation by autistic people allows for a real dialogue between autistic people and those who could benefit from understanding them. Programs like this are quite small, and their impact has not been even close to fully realized yet, but non-stigmatizing training of this kind can help improve relationships.

Autism and jobs information are also often provided by many mainstream autism organizations, whether from the autistic or autism communities. In Canada, organizations such as Kerry's Place,[23] Autism Ontario,[24] and the Canucks Autism Network,[25] which was founded by the co-owners of the Vancouver Canucks hockey team, all offer employment programs for autistic adults. In the United States, organizations like the Autism Society of America also offer resources about employment.[26]

While these programs can be useful tools to get information about trends, it is hard to know exactly how to handle an autistic employee or how to work with an autistic employer because everyone is different. Therefore, patience and understanding are especially essential to understand any autistic person.

Employees and employers of all kinds make mistakes and may not even be right for their jobs. An autistic person can be ill-suited for a job, but so can a neurotypical. The difference for employers hiring an autistic person is that if the person is qualified for the job, they will be giving them the roots for something they may not have received much of in their lives: confidence, independence, and trust.

Given the unemployment rate of autistic people and the traumas associated with their experiences, providing them with the ability to prove they are good at something can change their lives.

## Public Education

Some readers may look at public education and say this has to do with children, not autistic adults. But as established elsewhere, whether an autistic person feels understood and respected or not starts young — usually most acutely in school. The same dynamics that happen with children at elementary and high school also follow adults into their lives after school.

Teachers and their peers still lack understanding as to how autistic people learn, including from what is often called the "unwritten curriculum," or the lessons in school that people learn outside of class instruction.

Some progress has been made here, as in the rest of society. Since the advent of education disability legislation, there has been an increased appreciation for people with learning disabilities. For example, Individualized Education Programs (IEP) were introduced. These have been criticized in many ways, including for being too generalized and not individualized enough. Nevertheless, they do offer services for students with disabilities to get the assistance they need within a regular school and helped integrate autistic people into mainstream schools.

Negative perceptions by other children and even staff are still a big part of school life for autistic children. In adulthood, the aftermath of mistreatment in school can be deeply lowered self-esteem, persistent anger, and a distrust of others, which even well-meaning neurotypical adult peers can be slow and sometimes unwilling to try and understand.

These perceptions also come in when talking about punishment, either from teachers or parents. In North America, it is common for teachers to give students a time out or detention when they are acting out and misbehaving; in adulthood, this can be a paid leave or suspension, if not a firing, from work.

Such punishments can be a problem for autistic people, of any age, especially when they are not accompanied by a clear explanation of what they did wrong. *If they do not understand what they did, they will not change.* In fact, an autistic person can feel persecuted if they feel like they are punished for no reason, and the problems can get worse. *It is always important to tell them explicitly.*

For instance, there could be a situation where an autistic person may have an extreme reaction, like saying something abusive to a person teasing them, or by throwing a tantrum. To one person, such as a boss or a teacher, what an autistic person might be doing is a totally unacceptable way of expressing anger. To that autistic person, however, it is the only way they can think of to get a person to stop annoying them. They might be doing it in a way that can reflect either immaturity or a prolonged period of real bullying that causes their patience to run out, but it's a way of standing up for themselves.

In this way, autistic and neurotypical people may have distinct thresholds and triggers, but they really are not so different from most other people in how they express anger. Of course, it is not acceptable to express anger this way. However, the motives for an autistic person acting like this and a neurotypical person doing this differ because they have dissimilar brains. *Treating them as the same is likely to lead to different outcomes, which is why each case must be handled differently.*

This can be hard for their peers to understand. An autistic person being treated differently can lead to resentment, and the politics involved may lead a boss to make a decision that is not in the best interest of the autistic person.

There is also the matter of how autistic people's intelligence is perceived. As covered before, they can be intellectually disabled geniuses, or more often somewhere in between. Whichever, their learning profile will be unique because of the varied level of skills they have in different areas.

This can cause confusion from teachers, or bosses, or other children, or co-workers. It may lead them to wonder what can be expected of that autistic person. Difficulties in areas of weakness can be mistaken for lack of effort, although an autistic person is trying but may not have the mental resources to handle cognitively or emotionally a task at a given time.[27] The nature of autism is that some days it is more possible to do some things than others.

With this as a setup, what can be done to help autistic children, who often take these written and unwritten lessons into adulthood, be better understood and be better able to manage the lessons of school?

One proposed approach is the "universal design for learning," which has been promoted by autistic advocates such as T.C. Waisman.[28] This is a curriculum designed with the widest range of people in mind, including those with disabilities. As advocates note, the name "universal" can be misleading. The program proposes a diverse curriculum that has something for everyone but may not be taught equally to everyone.[29] As this applies to autistic people, allowing them to focus on special interests can be one way to approach their education, though there are many different ideas for how to create a universal curriculum.

Rather than impose a curriculum that teaches subjects an autistic person might be abnormally disinclined towards, they may wish instead to tailor a course to a special interest. The belief is that autistic people will get more out of their education when it is customized more to their individual learning style than trying to force them to adapt to the normal curriculum. This is where the universal design for learning goes beyond current individualized programs in schools today. Current IEP programs do not alter the curriculum, just the ways that children can learn within it.

Tony Attwood, like other clinical psychologists who do not explicitly favour this idea, nevertheless has noticed this tendency in his own practice. He seems sympathetic to allowing at least some autistic people to use this approach: "They [autistic clients] say, 'what you're teaching me is a waste of time,' and it is. But they want to know about their special interest."[30]

This approach has detractors. Other approaches favour viewing an autistic person as someone who can do whatever other kids can do. This can involve having them do the same kinds of rote learning from a regular curriculum, with extra help necessary to deal better in a conventional classroom. The thinking is that a person will be happiest if they can do well on the same terms as everyone else.

As recently as the 1980s, this approach would have been called progressive. In a time when autistic people would have either been removed from society or expected to do well or not like everyone else in a regular classroom, the idea of having autistic children taking the same classes as everyone else eventually became accepted as the norm.

As more autistic people became visible, and as more supports were given, the educational prospects of autistic people started to improve.[31] It is an improvement on only the most meagre earlier education, but it is nevertheless an improvement both socially and academically for autistic people to be part of society.

Can the universal design for education be used to improve this model? Perhaps. The usefulness of a new idea is only as good as how it's put into practice.

Then there is the role of special education, which can provide useful education to children with particular needs, but which can also be a place where these kids can be seen as castoffs.

The 2007 Bollywood movie *Taare Zameen Par*, about a young boy with dyslexia named Ishaan who struggles through mainstream schools, shows this attitude well in art. Ishaan ends up getting properly taught by a teacher who comes from the special education system, where he sees this frequently.

Special education in public schools is most often conducted in self-contained classrooms, which means there is one teacher who teaches all subjects. While special education classrooms are often full of dedicated staff, and can have a purpose, they have also had their critics, particularly in the way they can be seen to isolate students and treat them prematurely as failures.

Julia Bascom, the executive director of ASAN as of this writing, discussed her experiences as an autistic person in special education on the *Uniquely Human* podcast. She believes this is a national American issue and not just her own issue.

> What really radicalized me was working in a self-contained special education classroom for a couple of years with middle school students — some of them had intellectual disabilities, some were presumed to have intellectual disabilities because they didn't have a good way to communicate. . . . Those students and I were very, very similar. They were expressed differently in some ways. But our experiences of the world and the ways our brains worked were very, very similar.
>
> But because I could talk most of the time, I was treated very differently [and was therefore put into a mainstream classroom]. . . . I was able to look at what my life would have been like had I been in one of these self-contained classrooms, which would have happened if my school district had followed the law at the time, and I would have been throwing a chair across the classroom too. A lot of the aides in this classroom really cared about these kids, but they were working in this very flawed system.[32]

While self-contained classrooms do have issues, some forms of special education do have positive outcomes. Some education tailored specifically towards autistic people, such as TEACCH, has had a measured positive effect on the outcomes for these kids.[33]

There are also problems that public education cannot solve. This usually goes deeper than the public education system can get into. Often, the most success in dealing with autistic people is at a level even more meaningful and intimate than through public education.

## Family

The most intimate level of public understanding for autistic people is in their family, both the ones they are born into and the ones they make with partners.

Parents of autistic children, especially if they're neurotypical, are sometimes baffled by their children, in both their strengths and their weaknesses. For Joan Callanan, a woman in her sixties from Massachusetts who has an adopted autistic adult daughter named Brianna, that occurred when her daughter was a teenager, after she was diagnosed. "I broke my wrist and had three surgeries, and she responded by saying 'I know how you feel, I broke my finger,'" she said. "I want to say that's a selfish statement, but what she's trying to say is 'I can relate to you.'"

Stories like this are common among parents like Joan. Autistic people can be jarring in their routines, personal preferences, and how they communicate. To express mild frustration, they can say something that sounds deeply disturbing. They can be completely indifferent to outside temperatures but find the temperature of shower water completely intolerable. Sometimes these patterns don't seem to make sense, and the difficulty can be compounded by an autistic person not communicating likes and dislikes in clear language.

Trying to decipher what an autistic person is trying to say can sometimes require prolonged careful attention. Each one is different, and by the time they are adults, they will also have developed differently. A late talker can become amazingly fluent by adulthood, for example.

Most parents hope that by the time their child is an adult, they will have understood how to communicate with them better and, where required, know how to take care of them.

There is a common trajectory for people who get to know autistic people well. The first step is the reaction to an autism diagnosis. This can vary widely between parents. In many cases, they are completely unsurprised by an autism diagnosis as they were the ones who asked questions first, or even because they themselves are on the spectrum. Some adults are diagnosed after their children are because they see signs of themselves in their children.

But while there is also a "getting to know you" phase, how a neurotypical parent understands an autistic person at first and adapts can widely differ. One response can be a much greater degree of acceptance. If the parents have enough knowledge to ask questions and learn, and especially when there is a common family trait, it can lead to a closer bond between the child and the parent.

Yet these relationships are not necessarily kumbaya. Even in an accepting family, accessing services and dealing with the more challenging aspects of autism can be a source of extra attention and frustration for the parents, as well as a source of difficulty in the child's life. Anger from this can become an issue in the house in general.

As Tony Attwood shows, even clinicians have noticed this:

> The enforced proximity of two inflexible and dominating characters with Asperger's syndrome can lead to animosity and arguments. The non-Asperger's syndrome partner and parent becomes an experienced diplomat, trying to "keep the peace" and facing problems of conflicting loyalties. Having two people with Asperger's syndrome in the same family can be like having two magnets — they either attract or repel each other.[34]

In a family with multiple autistic generations, the shared traits they understand can also be those that cause each other grief. A real personal difference, combined with a non-neurotypical way of identifying and dealing with emotions, can be a recipe for a lot of pain. Most often, they can have a mix of good times and bad, just like most families.

This is the case for Sheila Oakley, an autistic woman in her early sixties from Oregon, who has three autistic children, all in their thirties. They were given official diagnoses within a couple of years. Oakley said that while their family has issues just like any other, their autism diagnoses formed a bond and answered many questions they had about themselves for their whole lives. "It [having a label of autism] doesn't bother any of us," she said. "For all of us, it was just a validation . . . there's an actual reason why we're different."

Some parents can go on a journey: from believing at first that autism is a tragedy, and then coming to accept an autistic child, and then even going on to embrace autism.

Ray Richmond may not say that his son's autism is something to embrace, but now he at least doesn't view it as something to deny or run away from. He even sees that it has positives that should be accepted and nurtured. "I always viewed autism as akin to mental retardation, even though that's a term we don't use anymore," he said. "Now, I've seen that there are all kinds of people, with all kinds of abilities, all kinds of functioning under the umbrella of autism. I see it now more as a challenge that can be overcome."

Other parents can be resentful and stay in denial or non-acceptance for a long time. This group usually has bad outcomes. Unsurprisingly, autistic children who are raised by parents who do not accept them are more likely to experience adverse childhood trauma, which increases their chances of heart disease and mental health issues. This attitude also works against the parents. Those who accept their kids are themselves more likely to have positive mental health outcomes.[35] Parents who struggle to accept their autistic children should keep this in mind.

Just as meaningful to autistic people as their parents' reaction is that of their siblings. Relationships between them and their siblings can have extra layers of complexity, whether or not the sibling is also autistic.

People can have a mix of views towards their autistic siblings, as noted by Mary Van Bourgondien, a professor from TEACCH, in Fred Volkmar's compendium on autistic adults.

> Several studies report no adverse effects of having a sibling with autism. Despite the communication, social, and behavioral challenges associated with a diagnosis of autism, some children who have a sibling with autism endorse both admiration for and satisfaction with their brother or sister with autism. However, others report a lack of closeness and loneliness, a limited number of interactions within the family and with their siblings in

> particular, and thoughts that their sibling with autism is a burden in comparison to the typical siblings of children with other disabilities.[36]

All siblings can have contentious relationships with each other, but there are some unique dynamics and challenges with an autistic sibling. Some complain about the lack of attention they receive from their parents because of the attention their autistic sibling requires, or at least gets.[37] This can be because they are often competing for attention and, especially later in life, resources. Sometimes an autistic person, who may not have the social skills, intelligence, or confidence to stand up for themselves, can fall prey to a jealous sibling who may be looking to take advantage of them or get something from their parents that may be theirs.

In general, as Van Bourgondien says, such difficulties do not appear to be the norm. Many autistic and neurotypical siblings have normal or even abnormally close relationships, which can help provide a source of support for an autistic person's entire life.

Some of the reasons this may be the case are more public awareness in general and sibling support groups in autism organizations. There is an Autism Sibling Support program at the Organization for Autism Research, for instance.[38] This American-based non-profit provides public access and help with research literature and other services. In Canada, there are also specific sibling supports at Kerry's Place's All About You program.[39] Broader sibling support, such as the Sibling Support Project,[40] an organization that began in 1990, offers programs for siblings of people with disabilities in general.

There are the ways autistic people are perceived by their family, and then there are ways autistic people are perceived as parents and family creators themselves.

This is a particularly sensitive topic, as people with disabilities of all kinds were historically thought to be unfit to have children. The efforts of eugenics programs to sterilize this group, as well as people with disabilities in general, are well-documented in many countries worldwide.[41] A report from the National Women's Law Centre in 2019 also said that forced sterilization of people with disabilities is still legal in thirty-one U.S. states.[42]

Thankfully, the days dramatized by *I Am Sam*, when a person like Sam was questioned for his ability to parent his daughter based on his autism, are largely over. There is still a stigma around autistic parents, but it's not acceptable to discriminate against autistic people wanting to have children. In the disability activist community, this is sometimes called the "right to procreate."[43] Eugenics is now a dirty word. This is a welcome change. At no other time in human history were autistic parents thought of this way.

There are special challenges to being an autistic parent. Evidence shows that some parents may need extra help to deal with the challenges, including some studies that suggest autistic mothers may need extra support.[44] Autistic people, however, are not inherently unfit to be parents.

The downsides of autism in parenting are probably readily apparent to many neurotypicals. Conventional emotional reciprocity can be seen as an issue, for example, as one person may feel they are not being given love and affection, even when it really is there but just expressed differently. While true, this is also as much a function of personality as it is of autism. Cold parents can be neurotypical or autistic.

The upsides, or at least the fun idiosyncrasies, are less well-documented as well. This has been noticed by clinicians like Tony Attwood who have particularly seen how this relationship can work when both the parents and child are autistic.

> There can be a natural bond, or antagonism, between a parent and a child who both have Asperger's syndrome [note: this book was written before the DSM-5 change]. Liane Holliday Willey [an autistic author who wrote *Pretending to Be Normal*] has a very close and supportive relationship with her father. He recognized that his daughter would need to acquire the knowledge he had learned about people, socializing and conversations. He became her social mentor, with daily advice on what to do and say in social situations. Father and daughter understood and respected each other's perspective and experiences.[45]

Relationships with parents are as important as relationships with significant others, if an autistic person decides they want one. Romantic relationships are more difficult to get into and maintain for autistic people on average.[46] This is often because many strangers, which all potential dating partners start as, can be inclined to dismiss someone who shows autistic characteristics — at least at first. Again, to their minds, it is not because they are autistic per se, it is because they are different and weird.

For this reason, autistic people sometimes restrict their dating to other autistic people, who are more likely to understand them. This can develop as a pattern, or it can happen because of a conscious choice.

"It's just more likely we'll make partners and friends with people who think like us," said Kira Trinity Gray. "I pretty much have only dated autistic people, without realizing it."

One positive about dating other autistic adults is that some traits do not require much explanation. However, just because two people are autistic does not mean they will get along.

The most important thing to look for from a potential romantic partner, neurotypical or autistic, might be whether they are understanding and curious or not. A certain open-mindedness is often needed when being with an autistic person in any way, but especially when dating. Autistic people are not a project, but they are different in ways that could use understanding and learning over time.

That is certainly the opinion of Brianna Callanan. "It's about finding the right person who understands," she said. "My boyfriend didn't know much about autism, but when we got together, he looked it up and got more information, so he'd be more aware and try to be more empathetic and understanding of my situation."

Just as in situations with a teacher or a parent, a romantic relationship can have the usual types of problems. A common one is that a neurotypical believes they are not getting enough affection because an autistic person does not say "I love you" enough or give them a hug. To an autistic person, saying "I love you" all the time can be redundant and pointless, giving them a hug can be uncomfortable, and the way they express connection is through enthusiastically showing their partner something about their special interest, which a neurotypical partner might not share.

It is extremely difficult to change the fundamentals of how a person thinks. However, these kinds of problems can be dealt with when autistic people and neurotypicals talk through their expectations and make time for them to be fulfilled.

Even if change on either side is difficult, it is often worthwhile. The neurotypical in the relationship broadens their experience of the world through seeing autism, while the autistic person, who may be in their first intense relationship, has their worldview opened by a deeper level of human connection.

What is shown at this level is that even the people who love an autistic person the most, who are the most exposed to them, can sometimes have difficulties with perceiving their needs. If this group has difficulty, the rest of society likely will as well.

## Conclusion

Public perception is increasing in both the number of people who know about autism and the percentage who think about it positively. It's much better to be autistic today than it was thirty, fifty, or one hundred years ago.

But there is still a lack of understanding of how autistic people can present, and why they do what they do. This can cause many people to see autistic people not as "different" or even better "autistic," but "weird" and therefore not to be dealt with.

Any individual autistic person's self-esteem should not be solely determined by how society views them. Because autistic people will always be different, they will likely always have some people who fear or dislike them.

There is no utopia where every neurotypical person completely understands and knows how to treat autistic people. Human beings notice differences, and sometimes they will be turned off by them.

However, a reasonable long-term goal can be that treatment by neurotypical people gets to a point where it can sometimes be a challenge to be autistic, but it is not a significant factor affecting their life outcomes. Current rates of suicide, educational and job attainment, and coexisting health conditions associated with autism, but not directly to do with autism, are evidence that society can do better.

At least some of these issues have to do with the loneliness, abuse, and rejection that come with negative public perception of "weird" people.

Like anyone else, autistic people must find foundations to their self-worth that are not dependent on the approval of others. Also like all humans, they are affected by them. This intersection is the subject of what is likely the most enigmatic and essential part of the autistic experience.

# CHAPTER 8:
# AN ISSUE OF SELF-UNDERSTANDING

FOR MOST AUTISTIC PEOPLE, struggling to be understood by others is often related to the struggle to understand themselves.

The earliest autistic autobiographers of the 1980s and 1990s, from Temple Grandin to Donna Williams, were trying to promote a greater public understanding of autism when they first wrote their books. It was also clear throughout their writing that they were also trying to discover themselves.

This is an essential part of the autistic experience, as well as perhaps the hardest and most meaningful.

Life is different when you do not feel difference. Neurotypicals live in a world where their basic social rules and cognitive expectations are shared by most other people, and where their social understanding and experience of the world is generally not a barrier to love, work, and friendship. They may know what it is like to be different in other ways, but not this way.

When most of the world fits with a person's assumptions, it is the differences that they notice. The choice is whether to explore these differences, ignore them, or stigmatize them. Stigmatizing and ignoring can be easy options — they do not have to think about their own sameness if they don't want to.

Autistic people, by contrast, see a world of differences from birth. Their way of existing is not "different" to them, as everyone's subjective experience is familiar to that person. But they do not have a choice except to understand neurotypicals unless they want to be social outcasts. This fundamentally affects how they see the world.

As social creatures, humans often believe that being in a minority means you are likely to be wrong or, as is often the case with autistic people, weird and damaged. This can be frustrating for autistic people, because as Donna Williams once wrote, "inside my head, what I was doing was completely sane."[1]

At least some of how people form their self-image is by what others tell them they are. Many autistic people have a constant war in their minds between the validity of their own perceptions and what other people think of them. Although they may know that they can do intellectual tasks others can't, their social naïveté and other weaknesses might lead others to dismiss them as stupid.

If that autistic person is in an environment where they are repeatedly told they are stupid, does that person then view themselves, at least fundamentally, as smart or stupid?

Autistic people can also get both positive and negative messages from the culture. Sometimes one wins out over the other; there can also be a war of contradictions.

This is where the idea of culture comes in. Being autistic has often been compared to being an "anthropologist from Mars," as the British scientist Oliver Sacks once wrote, quoting Temple Grandin.[2] If a person was taken up in a spaceship and put onto another planet, or even on a plane to another culture, their surroundings and expectations would suddenly become quite different and difficult to navigate.

While foreign cultures are fascinating, and over time a person may learn to fit in, it is a significant struggle to live in one. Culture shock over the long-term is a profound experience for many people who live outside their own, just as it is for an autistic person trying to understand the world.

But autistic people have no other planet to go to. Their disconnection is based on what is inside their brain, not their environment. There is no country where autistic people can go to that will not make them different.

Also, unlike culture, autism is also more hardwired and sometimes much more extreme in its differences, and the people from the host culture may also see a foreigner as a curiosity and understand their mistakes, at least to a degree, not as a "weird person" to be avoided.

In a standard debate about immigration, for instance, there is usually a question about whether to allow immigrants to maintain their old cultures or push them to assimilate. This is also a significant debate among people interested in autism. The question in this world is also how much society should accept autism, and neurodiversity in general, and how much autistic people should "assimilate" — as much as that's even possible.

If there is any concession towards assimilation, the question then becomes: How does an autistic person try to assimilate without betraying who they really are? The assumption behind this question is that autistic people, like almost all people, have a core personality that is essential or desirable. Giving that up would cause a massive existential crisis, and therefore shouldn't be contemplated.

The increased understanding of autism in the last thirty years also adds a completely new dimension to this question. Almost all people know they are part of a culture and going from one to another is going to be steep a learning curve.

However, not all autistic people knew they were autistic. Before Lorna Wing, and especially before Leo Kanner, they were diagnosed as "schizophrenic" or given even more common and judgmental terms: defective, antisocial, immature, or not properly brought up. They certainly did not exist even as different, never mind as a distinct culture like those with other disabilities, such as deaf and blind people. Autistic people existed as a group of broken neurotypicals, and when those "cultural" differences were revealed, they were rejected and did not know what was wrong with them.

While all autistic people understand this, there is a whole generation of them that understands more than anyone else.

## Lost Generation

When there is a big change, there will be those familiar with the old world and those young enough to only know the new one. The autistic community is now like this.

Autism researchers, most notably Simon Baron-Cohen, have written about a "lost generation." This term refers to people born before 1980, roughly, who have fundamentally different experiences of autism than those who were born since.[3] This is because of the addition of an autism diagnosis in the DSM-III published in 1980. The rate of diagnosis especially opened with the labels reflecting Wing's autism spectrum, like PDD-NOS, childhood developmental disorder, and Asperger's syndrome. People born before 1980 could not have received these diagnoses as children, which left a gaping hole that was filled by the autism diagnosis in those fortunate enough to get one. Without the diagnosis, there were less accurate and flattering ways to fill the void.

"Nobody ever said I had autism, I was just weird," Christina Linwood, an autistic New Zealander, said with a laugh. Linwood, showing how public perception can impact self-perception, was born in 1977.

Most people born before 1980 who would receive a diagnosis today would not have when they were children. People born before 1980 also had the risk of being institutionalized, reflecting a world where to be autistic was officially seen as being damaged. Being autistic before the DSM recognition was not just socially undesirable, it could even put a target on people's backs by powerful institutions, so it was seen as a serious problem to be labelled that way.

Michael John Carley, for instance, was "merely" assessed to have "emotional disturbance due to death of father" during a childhood school evaluation in 1973. He understands full well what this meant in retrospect, as stated on the *Uniquely Human* podcast, which like the book, is also a creation of Barry Prizant. "Back then, if anything like an autism diagnosis had been placed on me, I would have been sent to a home perhaps," he said. "I'm very grateful that they screwed up and mistook my behavioural differences for my father's death in Vietnam."[4]

A stark feature of this generation is a perpetual feeling of confusion and an inability to get answers for why their life was so hard. This is because they would have been dealing with real differences in their brain but would have had no medical reason to believe they were anything other than "weird" or "alien."

It's hard to exactly quantify the toll it took on people of this generation. Anecdotal accounts suggest that this experience was traumatic for many of them.

"I had such a hard time [as a kid] so I tucked things away," said Jasmin van Praet, an autistic woman in her early forties from Belgium.

> I don't have many active memories as a child. I was the oddball, and I really tried to fit in, and sometimes I managed for a little while, but I never truly nailed it. I would be bullied, and I never knew what I did. I would be in relationships that would end, and I never knew why. . . . It weighs on you.

Van Praet added that she believes in the strengths of diagnosis, because it helps you "figure out who you are."

Almost all people are familiar with this part of the human experience, often felt most acutely in adolescence, as noticed by psychologists like Erik Erikson.[5] For autistic people, the experience is especially complicated. It can be about more than finding your identity, it can even be about finding your humanity.

If a person is led to believe they are strange and fundamentally different, this can effectively make them feel like they are an alien. When they discover they are just differently wired but not less of a human, it has important effects on their view of themselves. It changes how they perceive their past, present, and future. To use the old autism rights slogan, they are not defective; they are just different.

That is usually much easier to live with in terms of self-perception, especially when they find people with the same experience, which can often happen after a diagnosis. This can change their life. Suz Fisher compares finding out she was autistic to when she converted to Christianity. "It's that feeling of 'I've found my people,'" she said. "It was a truth that I never realized or processed before, and now I have."

Of course, this is merely one way to sum up the feelings that can come. Many who find out they're autistic describe it as a revelation, not as a religious experience. Thankfully, most autistic people now do not learn this when they are in middle age; therefore, they can at least know why they are different for most of their lives.

There is evidence that outcomes are better among the generation born after 1980 than the older one. Outcome studies are difficult to conduct because of changing criteria for autism, going from DSM-III, to III-R, to IV and now to DSM-5. There is also difficulty in defining subjective metrics like "good," "fair," or "poor," especially when comparing one study to another or over one time or another.

However, the broad consensus is that outcomes, defined by measures like being employed at their educational level, number and quality of friendships, and romantic relationships, have been getting better over time, reflecting that the progress of knowledge believed to have been made over the last thirty years has made an impact.[6]

A lot of why this is true is related to autistic people and their parents having this knowledge and being able to find beneficial ways of dealing with it, including services and accommodations that work much better than they did previously. At the very least, they are almost certain not to be put into institutions, which were prevalent before the 1980s.

According to Barry Prizant:

> There are many, many reasons why we see better outcomes . . . One of the reasons is early intervention . . . parents are better supported now than they ever were before, so there's much more carry over to the home environment. . . . Inclusion has gone up tremendously; there's good educational programs.
>
> I think augmented and alternative communication have made a big difference, because a major reason there might be a poor outcome is if the person doesn't have an effective communication system, because that leads to frustration, that leads to aggressive behaviour.

He also went on to say that combating societal ignorance, misunderstanding from employers, and also making the world more sensory-friendly are ways that adults' lives could still be made better. He is not wrong.

Prizant's views on these lessons are also shared by at least some younger autistic people, like Charlie Sansom. Being diagnosed before age five, he believes early intervention really helped alter the course of his life in a good way. "I don't believe I would be where I am today without it," he said.

Many autistic people of this lost generation, who are forty and above, are still alive, which means this subject still really matters. Whether or not they have a diagnosis, they will need special attention and care from their families and societal institutions, not just because of their age but because of their experiences. They will have been less likely to have had support from their families, friends, and employers because, during their formative years, far fewer people in their community and in broader society were likely to understand them.

An older autistic person may also be less able to understand and take care of themselves because they were not made aware of who they were early on and may not have approached life with this in mind. An autistic person who is younger is more likely to have had opportunities to get the attention and knowledge they need.

This generational misunderstanding is true not just for less obviously autistic people whose traits were overlooked but for more obviously autistic people whose traits were tragically misunderstood. In previous times, the latter group was more likely to be diagnosed and often institutionalized.

In many ways, their traumas were especially intense. More obviously autistic people may have been treated badly and not given the necessary care in institutions, where many went after families rejected them. The simultaneous rejection by their family and society can be particularly psychologically damaging.

Outside observers sometimes believe that a person with a profound disability does not understand what is happening around them. However, all people instinctively know when their needs are not being met, even if they cannot express it in conventional ways.

Even some people on the less obvious end of the spectrum were also institutionalized. In GRASP meetings with autistic adults, Michael John Carley saw many people who went through the institutionalization process. In his 2008 book, *Asperger's from the Inside Out*, which relates the experiences of many autistic people, the institutionalization stories stand out for the level of bitterness they felt.

> One young man, diagnosed at age twenty-four [note: this meeting was decades ago, which explains his young age], could not survive a single GRASP support group without passionately expressing anger toward his parents, or for the world that would not employ him or provide him with companionship. It's one thing to do this at one meeting, but it's another thing to repeat the tirade at subsequent meetings.
>
> He'd had a truly rough time. He had been mistakenly institutionalized by his parents in a residential psychiatric hospital when he was thirteen, and he stayed there for years, not only enduring the debilitating atmosphere and the loss of developmentally appropriate experiences, but also becoming harmed by misprescribed antipsychotic pharmaceuticals that contained damaging short-and long-term side effects.
>
> Now correctly diagnosed, but unable to handle all the mistakes that had transpired in the past, he was

> uncontrollably mired in anger. The rest of this particular GRASP group appealed to his very evident intellectual abilities, as well as to his particular faith (he was a very religious person) that he needed to let much of this go.[7]

The story sums up the anger that can be felt by the "lost generation" in general. However, this story means a lot for other reasons. The ability to forgive and let go of anger is associated with positive mental and physical health outcomes, and this story teaches neurotypicals about the unique challenges autistic people have faced, while also teaching a lesson to autistic people about healthy ways to cope with life.[8]

Research on older adults is still lacking, so it is difficult to truly understand their needs. *But if an older autistic person shows signs that they could be autistic, it is always a safe bet to treat them with particular attention and empathy.* They may have gone through an experience like the one Carley described.

As individuals, older autistic people will differ among themselves. Some even thrive due to their family's love or their own inner strength and ability to regain confidence against substantial odds. As a group, however, they have significant challenges: overcoming mistreatment in their childhoods, not having the tools to deal with these challenges as an adult, and if they are still alive today, likely dealing with complicated lives and a shortage of support from family and friends.

It should be emphasized that autistic lives are still constant in many ways. A disproportionate number of younger people on the spectrum still struggle despite all the gains made. Not all young people are diagnosed early, and not all of them do well even if they have a diagnosis.

The experiences of the "lost generation," including its youngest members who are barely middle-aged, show that basic self-understanding of who they are as an autistic person comes earlier to more autistic people now. Overall, this leads to less difficult and more fruitful lives.

Today, the goal is to continue the progress that has been made including working on new ways to identify autistic people at younger ages and with less stigma. While efforts to do so have succeeded across all demographics, some traits make such success more likely than others. This is one of the most top-of-mind issues both within and outside autistic circles.

## Minority Identities

For some autistic people, their identity issues are deeper than dealing with just autism and their coexisting conditions. There are racial, sexual orientation, and gender identities that exist within the autistic community that add another layer of complexity. This has only recently really started to get more attention among researchers and the public.

These identities have an impact on each other as well as on the individual. Many anecdotes and studies show how gender roles impact diagnosis, how cultural factors and racism affect how an autistic person is treated, and even whether being autistic means a greater likelihood of having these identities.

The transgender and gender non-binary community have been particularly visible recently for this reason. This is partly because of the increased prominence of this community in general, as well as the fact they represent a greater percentage of the autistic population than in the general population.[9]

There is still a large gap to be filled in researching this issue. Although this is a relatively newly discovered link, at a social and organizational level, the overlap between these communities has created a tight bond between them. It is unclear how much of this overlap is biologically or socially caused, but some autistic people suspect elements of the autistic community may be attractive to transgender people. This is not evidence of a causal link, but something that may explain why the two communities are close.

"We don't pick up on a lot of social signals, including gender expectation," said Michael John Carley. "Here's a real benefit to being so socially clueless. Because all that harmful stereotyping bypasses us and we're so much more conditioned to be in tune with how we feel and not what the rest of the world wants us to feel, especially about our sexuality and our bodies."

Rae Madrid, a Chicagoan over forty who is transgender and identifies as non-binary, only discovered they were autistic as an adult during the COVID-19 pandemic. But they provide a case study of how people can live with not just one but two complex identities in their minds.

The tell-tale signs of autism have been there from Madrid's childhood. Their stories, which include watching the same movie five times in a summer, wearing the same shoes even as they were falling apart, and taking non-literal speech literally, are all deeply relatable to many autistic people.

"When I was in high school, I got voted 'most likely to start a cult,'" Madrid said with a laugh, referring to how they were perceived as weird by others.[10] On top of their autism, Madrid's transgender identity goes back even longer, so they know what it felt like to be different even before they knew they were autistic.

The experience of being continually rejected based on even one unchangeable identity can be a life-defining wound for many people. This even bears out in health statistics, as rates of self-harm and depression for transgender people are worryingly high — far higher than in the general population.[11]

Some transgender people deal with this in a different way. It's not as if Madrid doesn't feel rejection, but their experience has led to them embracing a kind of radical self-acceptance, which means accepting everything about them that others may look down on. If a person has radical self-confidence, it can lead them to being radically accepting of others. With experience and understanding of themselves, autistic transgender people find beauty and acceptance in people that most of society finds bizarre.

"I'm sure that being rejected, partially for my autistic traits, led me to say 'fine, reject me, I'll just find acceptance within myself,'" said Madrid. "It leads me to be really open-minded about what can that look like."

This attitude helps when autistic people, as well as other minorities, meet up. Madrid agrees with Carley's view that autistic communities can be a place where the members' personalities meant they were more able to be themselves, and even to find out new things.

"When you learn that [you're different], you can just embrace your differentness," said Madrid. "I don't think being autistic makes someone be trans, it's just that you're more willing to find things out about yourself that they might otherwise repress."

Autistic spaces and even autistic people as a group have been written about where there is a reduced level of the kinds of prejudices that can exist in more neurotypical circles. There is controversy about how much this is true. Prejudices can exist among autistic people, as among any group, and some researchers have written about how this is true, if possibly reduced.[12]

One contributing factor to the overall reduced prejudice is the knowledge of what it is like to be different. This includes differences known to transgender people and more traditional struggles.

The struggle for autistic women goes back to when the understanding of autism began and is still strongly present and talked about in autism circles today. The good news is that women have been more visible in the public conversation about autism. Books such as *Aspergirls*, *Autism in Heels*, and *Spectrum Women*, all published since 2010, have started to change this perception that autistic people are "young cis boys," as is derisively said by some autistic self-advocates.

Fictional autistic female characters are also evident in popular media, whether for kids, like Julia from *Sesame Street*, or adults, like Detective Sonya Cross from *The Bridge*. These show autistic women exist for a popular audience who may not have otherwise considered them.

There has also been a rise in real-world activism relating to autistic women, sometimes intertwined with transgender activism. Some self-advocacy organizations are specifically dedicated to looking at non-cis-gender men, like the Autistic Women and Non-Binary Network.

It is still nevertheless true that autistic women have issues as a group. Though among the first autistic people to write about their experiences, they have historically been overlooked as a group by society and clinicians.

The most obvious place to start is the rate of diagnosis. Males currently outnumber females in autism diagnosis at a ratio of around 4:1.[13] This is virtually unchanged from Leo Kanner's estimate, which he gave as early as 1958.[14] In recent years, this has come into question. Some now claim the estimate may be 3:1 because of the number of women believed to be overlooked, and it could even be more than that.[15] This ratio also narrows considerably in cases of autism with traits of more obvious presentation, with a rate of 1.7 men to 1 woman when there is moderate to severe intellectual disability.[16] This group is also more likely to be diagnosed in general.

This difference, whether it is 4:1, 3:1, or 2:1, may reflect the fact that more men than women really are autistic. However, even if this is true, the percentage of autistic women represents a significant minority that still deserves being treated as an important and distinct subject.

Conversely, if there is a diagnosis rate among women below their actual numbers, it has negative impacts for many reasons, including the pain and suffering autistic women go through for which they have no explicable cause. As with diagnosis in general, if an autistic woman does not know they are autistic, they will have a much harder time getting the help they need.

This experience seems to be significantly more common in women than men. Even though the age of autism onset is the same for both, evidence suggests that women on average get diagnosed later than men.[17] It takes longer for the rest of society to recognize autism in women, which often can mean it takes longer for the women themselves to realize their difference.

Autistic adult women also deal with issues their male counterparts encounter less often, such as having their lack of social understanding taken advantage of by predatory men. This is reflected in significant rates of sexual assault against autistic women, higher than neurotypical women.[18] A woman who has difficulty reading social cues will be less aware of the tendencies of abusive men, and therefore more likely to be abused.

This increased vulnerability, as well as increased anxiety among autistic women, also contributes to their tendency to have worse outcomes than men on numerous metrics, like rate of sexual assault and mortality.

Then there are also gender stereotypes. Christina Linwood has experienced some of the ways that being an autistic woman can cause perception problems from others, even when it comes to people in her life talking about one of her prior relationships.

"Everyone says 'poor Tim,[19] poor Tim,'" she said. "He's such a dependable bloke, and he has to put up with crazy Christina who is so demanding of people and such a nightmare to be around." The man was seen as more level-headed than her by people around her, even though she explained that he was really an unpleasant and abusive person.

Linwood, who works in information technology, is an example of a person who is resilient and knowledgeable. However, she has had difficulty fitting in at times in her life — not just due to her autism but particularly how others view a woman with autism. The people in her life may not even consciously see it that way. Many are not knowledgeable enough about autism to understand it on its own, never mind how it interacts with gender. There's a strong case, however, for a unique intersection between autism and gender to be there if a person knows what to look for.

Some theoretical research has given validity to the existence of this gap. Simon Baron-Cohen wrote in his 2004 book, *The Essential Difference,* about the "extreme male brain."[20] What he meant by this was the differences between men and women, as groups, with traits he called "empathizing" and "systemizing."[21] Women, broadly, are "empathizers," while men, broadly, are "systemizers." This refers to the tendency for women to be interested in people, while men are interested in the physical world.

These traits have been attributed to broad gender differences. They include what kinds of careers each choose, as men are more likely to be engineers and women to be nurses, and what personality traits are more common, such as who is more likely to express affection and how they do it.[22]

Baron-Cohen said that autistic people had an "extreme male brain," in that he believed a core trait of autistic people was that they were extreme systematizers.[23] Where this relates to women and autism is that seeing extreme levels of these traits in males could be viewed as odd, but not extremely atypical, and therefore less likely to be regarded with as much skepticism and hostility. By contrast, since women are expected to care more about people, they may be seen as especially odd if they care more about the physical world, and the social pressures can be particularly difficult as a result.

The "extreme male brain" idea is a controversial one. This might be expected given the contentious nature of sex and gender issues. Even if people see females having more traditionally "male" interests, it may help to explain why autistic women can get unique stigmas attached to them. Because of this stigma, among other possible reasons, a female autistic person's traits may also be hidden more often. Autistic women have long been speculated to hide their traits even by clinicians. As Tony Attwood said, if a girl makes a social mistake, they may apologize and everyone else moves on, whereas a boy is more likely to make a scene.[24] This makes it more probable that the boy will be referred and diagnosed, though some autistic people think the story goes deeper.

"For all the recent media coverage of camouflaging, I sense it's become a buzzword and a victim-blaming excuse for systemic failures," said Angeline Adams, an autistic woman in her thirties from Northern Ireland. "'Of course, we're not managing to diagnose girls; they camouflage!' And these are often children who are having sensory overload, meltdowns, self-harming."

The literature on camouflage and the difficulty with measuring this, as covered in chapter 5, makes this hard to verify scientifically. However, it is a widely held hypothesis that has a lot of interest and one that many autistic women can relate to.

"Ask a kid, I learned to mask very young," said Sara Luntz, an autistic woman based in the Western United States. "I just kept everything in."

Even at the low estimates, more males than females are believed to be autistic, which helps explain the disproportionate attention by researchers, service providers, and the public towards males in the autism world. The evolving nature of the knowledge of autism means it may include many more females than previously understood.

Autism has the same broad criteria for diagnosis, but because men and women differ biologically and socially, they may express it differently. This should be much more broadly comprehended by everyone: educators can identify girls who may need extra help, parents can recognize traits in children, and researchers can better understand autism in girls.

The most important people who should pick up this message are autistic women themselves. Right now, they are less likely to be recognized as autistic by others, so the hope in the future is that they can identify their differences and communicate to others that their pain and struggle reflect autism, not brokenness.

Sex and gender are not the only identities that connect to autism. Members of ethnic minorities are another example of having to untangle two identities. For complex cultural and socioeconomic reasons, white people in North America have historically been diagnosed at greater rates than non-white people.[25] This affects perceptions of autistic people who are ethnic minorities not just in the wider society but also within their communities. As already shown, increased familiarity improves attitudes towards autistic people, which also helps to show differences in attitudes between Black, Asian, and white autistic people. The perception of autism was better among white Americans than Black and Asian Americans.[26]

This likely reflects how the rates of diagnosis differ between these groups. This is useful when figuring out why it is important to increase diagnosis in ethnic minority groups. It is not just about a relationship with the wider society, as racial issues are often rightly discussed, it also helps autistic people within their own families and other people within their ethnic group.

This whole topic has only recently started to gain attention. In 2017, *All the Weight of Our Dreams* was published which was centred on a neurodiversity point of view through multiple writers. Among them were Lydia X.Z. Brown and Morénike Giwa Onaiwu, who are also members of the Autistic Women and Non-Binary Network.[27] It featured interviews, personal essays, and poems written by Black, Asian, and other non-white autistic people. Literature on race and autism, whether in the academic or popular world, is still relatively rare, and vignettes like this therefore offer valuable insight from at least one Black autistic perspective.

> I am raising Black children, autistic and non-autistic. I am already afraid for them. My oldest son, a teenager, is soon going to be too old for the bubble of protection that comes with youth — and will have to face life as one of the most difficult things to be in this country: a Black male. But my 3-year-old son — my sweet, kind, fun-loving youngest child — will have to face life as male. And Black. And autistic. What will that mean for him? That he will be viewed as a violent, only half-human individual that doesn't deserve to exist because aside from being "flawed," he's also a danger?[28]

The political slant of much of the book, which is quite strongly left-wing, may make the contents objectionable to some readers. Nevertheless, it is a rare attempt to chronicle the autistic experience through the writings of autistic minorities. Its example should be followed — more of this is needed.

On one level, there is being in a minority, and then on another, living in a country where services for autistic adults are not as developed as they are in countries with stronger economies. Autism is a global human trait that affects all ethnicities and nationalities. In the developing world, however, it is less considered than it is in more economically prosperous countries. There, rates of diagnosis tend to be higher, and there is more education, services, and professional understanding.

Sudhanshu Grover said that, in her home country of India, getting paperwork needed to access services can be difficult because diagnosis is still much more of a problem due to a lack of understanding about the full breadth of what autism can be.

"Awareness has gone up hugely... but acceptance not so much [in India]," said Grover. "People with more subtle presentation are hugely misunderstood. It's mostly up to them for getting services. You need a certificate to get services, and this is extremely challenging if you have more subtle presentation."

Of course, this is a common problem worldwide, but in India, where the rate of autism diagnosis is 0.23% of the population, compared to 1.47% in the United States, there is still a long way to go.[29] The situation in India is likely true generally for regions outside of developed Western and Far East Asian countries.

As is true in many societies regarding race, gender, and sexuality, discussions of "privilege" also exist within the autistic community. It is not uncommon to hear about autism's historical connection to "upper-middle-class cisgender white boys below the age of ten," especially from people who never fit one or more aspects of this description. White male children are also often believed to be represented more in public discussions about autism.[30]

This description contains some degree of truth. Autism as a concept known today was discovered in European countries and North America. Many of Kanner and Asperger's earliest patients fit something like this description. For instance, Donald Triplett's mother's education and personality, which were much more evident among the upper middle class of Kanner's time, were noted in his writings.[31]

Many of the earliest pioneers of autism research were not unlike the class and race identifiers outlined, though the gender of the researchers is much more mixed. Researchers sometimes worked in male and female teams: Beate Hermelin and Neil O'Connor, Hans Asperger and Sister Viktorine, and Bernie Rimland and Ruth Sullivan, just to name a few. This is likely also influenced by the psychology profession being more predominantly women.[32]

To this day, white males, especially from relatively well-off families, are still more likely to be diagnosed. As a group, they are likely to be luckier, in that they are more apt to get diagnosed early and, therefore, to get services relating to autism, and this should be acknowledged.[33]

Consequently, there should be greater awareness of women, transgender and non-binary people, and minorities, and greater attempts should be made to identify and help them.

It should also be emphasized that autism is still autism regardless of race, sex, gender and sexual orientation. If there are three autistic people in a room — a white male, a Black female, and an Asian non-binary person — they may have some differences based on other identities, but they will all have stories about the social difficulties, personal quirks, and heightened senses that are common traits. This identity alone unites many people, and this will be in addition to other aspects of their personalities they share that all make them human.

## Sexuality and Dating

In the popular TV show *The Good Doctor*, Shaun Murphy, an autistic savant who is a surgical resident in San Jose, is shown taking the bus and being interested in its risqué lingerie ads. This scene follows another where he talks to his colleagues Jared Kalu and Claire Browne, who are treating a young porn actress with a sexually transmitted disease. After being asked whether the actress was in the kind of porn that had stories, Kalu wonders out loud whether porn has storylines anymore. Kalu expresses surprise when Murphy interjects with "sometimes," implying he watches porn.

Kalu asks him, with evident surprise, whether he watches porn or not. Browne, who is established by this point in the show to be more understanding of Murphy, responds slightly condescendingly to Kalu, "He's a guy, all guys watch porn." Browne may as well have ended this sentence with, "including the autistic ones."

Kalu's comment is reflective of a popular misguided view that autistic people are not interested in romance or sex. While a few, like some neurotypical people, are asexual, there is nothing inherent that prevents them from being interested in dating or sex. This is implied in other sections of this book, such as those about online dating and relationships in general.

What is different is how their social, sensory, and emotional development allow autistic people to successfully flirt, date, and have sex, and how this aspect of their lives affects how they perceive themselves. While the data about how many of them are in relationships is unreliable, it is a safe assumption that rates of romantic relationships and marriage are a lot lower for autistic people than neurotypicals.

This is also one area where profiles of men and women can look quite different. Sarah Hendrickx, a British autistic woman and clinician famous for her writings about autistic girls, has said that autistic people can have their first sexual experiences later, even into their thirties and forties, but she particularly writes this about male clients.[34] Of course, this can range widely.

Given that men are more often expected to initiate sex, and that autistic men often have issues with self-confidence and anxiety, it may take more time for them to have the assurance necessary to date and be sexually active.[35]

By contrast, autistic women can begin sexual relationships about the same time as their peers — in their teens.[36] The danger in this is that young autistic women are particularly vulnerable because of their naïveté and lack of social skills. Therefore, they can be talked into doing sexual activities they do not want to do and be more vulnerable to abusive relationships in general.

The concern is not the existence of their sex lives, it's much more the quality of it. There's the quality of sexual experiences, then there is the quality of the way people think about sex. Michael John Carley, who wrote *The Book of Happy, Positive, and Confident Sex for Adults on the Autism Spectrum and Beyond* in 2021, started having sex in his teen years and had multiple partners before getting married.[37] However, as a member of the "lost generation," he was not diagnosed with Asperger's syndrome (as it was then called) until his late thirties.[38]

Carley has said that his defiance and confidence in his youth helped him overcome some of the traps that catch other autistic people, including in his sex life.[39] Having heard many autistic people speak in group sessions, he also understands how messages about sex can be interpreted by autistic adolescents and adults, which is often not how they are intended.

As demonstrated by Raymond Babbit, in *Rain Man,* when he justifies his refusal to fly based on listing airlines that have had planes crash (except Qantas, which apparently never crashed), how autistic people interpret information may not be how neurotypicals do. This can have unintended negative results.

Out-of-context and overly cautious education about sex is one of these ways, which can impact how autistic people view having the experience themselves.

"The thing that's so harmful in the autism world is that we're literal thinkers," Carley said on the *Uniquely Human* podcast.

> They would say, "I'm never going to have sex because I'm going to get an STD" "I'm never going to have sex because I'm afraid of having an unwanted pregnancy," or "I'm never going to look at a girl because I'm afraid of going to jail." . . . Our culture has done this to them, and it's so mean![40]

When autistic people make mistakes in dating their peers might not, like failing to discern whether someone is interested in them, it can fill them with a lot of anger. It can add one more factor to their poor self-image.

Unconventional development makes it challenging for autistic adults to understand themselves. Sexuality is no exception. An autistic person in their mid-to-late twenties may have little-to-no sexual experiences, or these were exploitative and abusive. Autistic adults were also more likely to be sexually abused as children.[41] Therefore, it can be harder to relate to other people on a sexual level.

When people are teenagers, everything about sex is new. In their twenties, they more commonly have a sexual history, which includes likes, dislikes, and expectations. People can expect their partners of comparable ages to have a similar maturity about sexuality, which an autistic person may not have yet developed. This can sometimes be a source of conflict in a relationship.

If autistic people are not getting sex, they can also retreat into places where there is a superficial sexual gratification, such as pornography. Too much porn use can be unhealthy, especially if it alters their views about what a healthy sex life is like. Tony Attwood is one of many clinicians who have written about this.

> If the teenager with Asperger's syndrome has few friends with whom she or he can discuss personal topics, such as romantic or sexual feelings for someone, the source of information on relationships may be television programmes ("soap operas" and situation comedies in particular) or pornography.[42]

However, anecdotes from clinicians are not necessarily representative of autistic people as a group. It is important to remember when reading clinical reports that they reflect people who are coming in to deal with problems. Clinicians report what they are seeing based on their own experiences with similar people. It doesn't consider the lives of people they are not seeing, and therefore should not automatically be assumed as typical.

This also does not mean most autistic adults are sexual perverts or have a total fantasy sex life; most do not. It only means that their challenges with sexuality are likely greater than for neurotypicals, who also use porn, including pathologically, and that the porn use may have an unintended effect that might not occur as much in neurotypicals because of how literally it can be taken as sex education.[43]

Autistic people can also have an unconventional approach to sexuality. This is not just a disproportionately high amount of identification with unconventional sexual labels, such as pansexual or asexual, but even with more familiar non-heterosexual identities.[44] As with the link with transgender people, most academic sources, such as books on autistic adults from researchers Susan Lowinger or Patricia Howlin, are not very detailed on gay people. Much more research is needed.

However, there are some things that are known. Autistic people have been reported to be more likely to identify as LGBTQ+ in general.[45] Although Lowinger's book says evidence exists that autistic women are more like to be attracted to other women, but autistic men are not more likely to be attracted to other men, it is not known why in either case.[46] However, the impact of being gay, whether male or female, as well as autistic makes their lives even more difficult in terms of discrimination and adversity, but also potentially less challenging.

It also makes it even more difficult to sort out an identity when there are two complex identities rather than just one, as well as two sources of discrimination from wider society. Both gay autistic men and women have reported safety issues when looking for partners and in ordinary life, just like gay men and women in general.[47] Autistic people, even if they are not gay themselves, may be more accepting of gay people because they are different to begin with and because autistic people may be more likely themselves to be gay. An autistic person, if they know other autistic people, can come out in their autistic community, where they will be less likely to be judged.

Gay relationships where one or both partners are autistic can also be highly supportive and a source of strength and support, as in any other.

"I've got a really good spouse, she really understands me," said M. "She took the trouble when I got the diagnosis to get books and read about what it really means to be autistic, so she's really supportive. She knows when I'm headed for meltdown and knows how to defuse my meltdown." M.'s story shows that all humans need support and attention. Autistic people need particular attention. This can help them avoid what can be the ultimate consequence of poor self-image.

## Mortality and Risk

Among researchers, there is a consensus that autistic people have at least some degree of excess mortality. Some claims based on isolated studies state that autistic life expectancy is around thirty-six or fifty-four,[48] but the exact age is unknown. Even basic data is in dispute, like the number of autistic people and their demographic makeup. Making reliable estimates on something more complex based on these kinds of measures is even more challenging. What *is* known is that autistic people, on average, die earlier.[49]

Autism itself is not believed to cause higher excess mortality. If an autistic person has their needs met and is in otherwise good health, they could live for as long as any neurotypical. Because of the world they live in, unfortunately, this is not the case.

The evidence suggests that many factors lead to excess early death in autistic people, including accidents and complications from seizures, which 10 to 40% of autistic people have, far higher than about 1% of the general population.[50] These are in addition to accidents in general, with two prominent kinds being drowning and suffocation.

Autistic children are also more likely to run away from their parents and be more unaware of danger, like running onto a busy street or outside in cold weather without winter clothes.[51] However, the worst outcomes from this only happen to a small minority of autistic children. This tendency also controversially leads to measures like putting "Autistic Child" warning signs on roads, which some parents see as protection, but others see as stigmatizing.

Autistic people are also at higher risk of heart disease, cancer, and drug overdose, all of which have lifestyle factors more common in autism that heighten the risk, like loneliness, bad diet, and trauma.[52] Evidence suggests that this is even more stark among women. A study published in 1998, which followed 11,347 people in California, looked at mortality rates among autistic people from 1980 to 1996. It showed that autistic women are at a 490% risk of early death compared to neurotypicals, compared to the 137% higher risk for autistic men.[53]

While it was not a definitive study, as criteria and diagnosis of autism were different especially for women at that time, it is thought-provoking. This is both because of the lifestyle factors that disproportionately impact women and girls and because life expectancy among neurotypical women is longer than for men.

The risk of suicide is sadly quite real and elevated among autistic adults. Though based on only a small number of studies, there is a consensus that suicide among autistic people is higher than in the general population.[54] Autistica, a U.K.-based autism organization, also has written that autistic people without a learning disability were nine times more likely to die by suicide. This challenges the "functioning" approach to autism.[55] The validity of this statistic is questionable considering what little is currently known. But it raises the concern of how autistic people who appear to be fitting in better can in fact be struggling.

This is also where mental and physical health often intersect. The increased risk of suicide and self-harm among autistic people is related to the increased risk of exclusion, bullying, and abuse. This risk can be measured in the form of adverse childhood experiences, which includes trauma inflicted by parents, peers, or non-family adults. At its greatest extreme, this also includes the relatively rare but sensational and tragic cases of caregivers, often parents, murdering the autistic people under their care.

The increased vulnerability to danger is sometimes known, either empirically or intuitively, to parents when they are raising their autistic children. This can lead to overprotection, which adds to the tension and anxiety those children can still feel as adults. They receive a message early in life that the world is a dangerous place. Moreover, this overprotection can also lead them to believe they cannot do anything for themselves.

In an ironic twist of fate, increasing vulnerability to anxiety makes them more prone to associated mental and physical health conditions, such as cardiovascular disease and depression, which can be fatal if untreated and too far advanced.[56]

Excess mortality can come from caring too much or caring too little, even in autistic people. Overprotection can create a sense of "learned helplessness," where autistic adults can believe that the safest way to operate in the world is to avoid doing things for themselves. This usually stems from being afraid or being overloaded with too much stimulation.[57] This can increase their problems with finding friends and romantic partners, getting exercise, or obtaining a job. The inability to handle the world on their own as much as they can makes them more vulnerable to the world, not less.

Likewise, the accident-related deaths can result from unfortunate incidents that are not anyone's fault but can also be related to caregiver negligence.

This leads to the most important aspect of the mortality discussion. It is not the death but the lifestyle patterns that helped cause it that ultimately mean something in real life. Death is caused not by autism but by the world around autistic people.

Mortality can result from complications of either negligence or overprotection; deaths are not just random and tragic. *Autistic people should be given the maximum amount of latitude within their capabilities.* The way any person would be treated should apply to an autistic person: if they have a history of dangerous risk-taking, they should be reined in; if a caregiver is restricting them from doing something they want to do that has normal risk, the caregiver should let go.

Autistic people, depending on their strengths and weaknesses, can do a lot of what a neurotypical person can. The risk involved to their self-image when they believe they cannot do anything right is potentially catastrophic to their functioning as an adult.

Knowing not to overprotect is not just for autistic people's happiness. Counterintuitively, loosening the reins can help them perhaps live a little longer too, if it means their happiness also reduces their anxiety and depression.

However, they may experience other health conditions, some of which have nothing to do with the outside world and seem to reflect being autistic, at least to some degree.

## Coexisting Conditions

The majority of autistic people have at least one coexisting physical or mental health condition. For example, the incidence of psychiatric conditions has been estimated as high as 86%, according to one study from Iran.[58]

Common psychiatric conditions more widespread in autistic people than the general population include attention deficit hyperactivity disorder (ADHD), obsessive-compulsive disorder (OCD), borderline personality disorder, and sleep disorders. Physical conditions more prevalent in autistic people include epilepsy, tinnitus, fragile X syndrome (a rare and disabling condition caused by DNA duplications), and tuberous sclerosis (where tumours grow in the brain and vital organs).

The first way these conditions help form a person's self-image is that they can make diagnosis more difficult. Given that an autism diagnosis is often a way for people to get clarity on who they are, a coexisting condition can make it more difficult to come to terms about themselves. They start to question whether their traits are related to them, their autism, or their coexisting condition.

If a young adult struggles academically because of their ADHD and socially due to autistic traits, this complicates how they view themselves and how others, including medical professionals, work with them. While it can be difficult for the doctors to untangle this, how the patients see this themselves is even more important. It can often take real resolve and effort to understand who they are and to do as well as they can, overriding societal and family stigmas about their other conditions in the process.

Although this harsh reality does not eliminate those conditions, these extra labels can help. For people like Andy H.,[59] a Colombian man now living in Canada, these extra diagnoses are like fitting together pieces of a puzzle. Autism does not necessarily explain everything a person experiences, but having these other labels can help solve unanswered questions. He said:

> I was diagnosed [after a medical leave from work] with attention deficit condition, autism spectrum condition, and obsessive-compulsive condition. They seem to summarize things I've faced in my life. . . . from attention deficit condition the lack of stability in jobs. . . . the OCD and ADD combined explain things in my life. I would say it's a relief, but at the same time now, I wouldn't call it a source of anxiety, but I know areas I need to address, and I'm working on those.

Among the many coexisting conditions prominent with autism, anxiety and depression deserve special attention. "What will always be with me is my anxiety," said Charlie Sansom, after talking about how his own health and autistic traits have changed since childhood. He is far from alone.

Autistic people have disproportionate rates of anxiety and depression compared to most people, which range widely depending on the study, with the lowest estimates around 22%.[60] Although this is not much higher than the National Institute of Mental Health's estimate of 19% in general, it's been shown as high as 39%, even in children, who are not expected to have high rates of depression.[61] While studies' estimates vary, these rates show a similar pattern. Almost everyone generally agrees that anxiety and depression rates among autistic people are at least somewhat significantly higher than neurotypical rates.

Clinical anxiety and depression are broad societal issues. These disabilities represent leading causes of lost time at work and negative physical health outcomes, not to mention suicide. This deserves to be taken seriously in any group of people, including autistic people.

In a more uncomfortable, unpredictable, and sometimes more hostile world, it is not surprising that autistic people would feel more anxious. Repeated failures and deficiencies in areas most others take for granted often make autistic people feel like the next failure is inevitable. They can also be slower to reach goals and milestones presupposed by their neurotypical peers, which can increase anxiety and depression.

This relationship is difficult to manage because of the stigma associated not just with autism but still with anxiety and depression, even if it is less so now than in the past. It is not uncommon for these disabilities, even in neurotypical people, to be discussed as if they were emotions the person could just control. This common misunderstanding is difficult for anyone struggling with clinical depression.

An autistic person, however, has a particular problem. What goes on in their head can sometimes be much more difficult for them to describe to others. Prolonged depressed mood because of a job loss or death in the family is relatively easy to explain, but depression because of them perseverating over memories most people would have long resolved, or having anxiety over socializing or sensory issues, can be particularly difficult to explain in a way other people will take seriously.

*Therefore, if someone who is autistic is showing signs of distress and low mood, it is best to be patient and try to understand an autistic person from their perspective.* Everyone has different thresholds and triggers, whether neurotypical or autistic, and trying to tell someone how they are supposed to feel usually isn't helpful.

Some of this has to do with a default expectation of many autistic people about how the world is supposed to work. An autistic person who takes certain moral principles in a completely literal and absolute way will be particularly affected when they see something that violates those principles. Their experiences of the world, including understanding that morality and day-to-day life is more relative and transactional for many others than it is for them, is often a jarring mismatch of expectations. This can be a factor in autistic people being depressed and skeptical of others. When both sides learn about how the other person sees these situations, it is easier for both people to have a stable, reasonable view of the world they can both live with.

There are also other traits that cause autistic people to be more likely to get depressed. A study published in the prestigious science journal *Nature* argued that alexithymia, a trait common in autistic people that makes it difficult to express and recognize emotions, was more of a predictor for depression than autistic traits themselves.[62]

Difficulty in understanding one's own emotions makes it challenging to understand oneself. As Tony Attwood said, in answering a question about mood with "I don't know," this often translates to "I don't know how to put all the feelings going on in my mind and put into speech that you'll understand."[63]

Many autistic people would relate to this experience, especially when they are overwhelmed. "I don't know" can mean they are experiencing the visceral sensation of being depressed, anxious, confused, and angry at the same time.

Being able to name the feeling people get in certain situations makes it easier to make emotional connections with others.

Finally, there is also a particularly sad coexisting condition possibly more common in autistic people — post-traumatic stress disorder (PTSD). The literature on this topic is still small, even for children. However, autistic people can have many more potential triggers for PTSD, such as vulnerability to physical and sexual abuse.[64] It frequently coexists with depression and anxiety, as well as other traits usually associated with autism, such as being withdrawn or perseverating on past events. This can make it especially challenging to diagnose because traits reflected by PTSD could also be autism, especially if traumas occurred in early childhood.[65] This correlation should be more studied as it can also lend insight into the lives of autistic people.

In addition, coexisting conditions, whether depression, ADHD, or others, are also commonly associated with drug use, both prescription and recreational. With autism thrown in, the picture becomes more complicated.

## Drug Use

For this section, the word "drugs" will encompass all legal and illegal mind- and body-altering substances, from nicotine to alcohol to opiates.

First are the legal kinds. There are only two FDA-recommended drugs specifically for autistic people: risperidone and aripiprazole, which were approved in 2006 and 2009 respectively. Both are meant to deal with irritability in children.[66]

However, there are also drugs to deal with common coexisting conditions. Some autistic people who have ADHD and are given drugs like Ritalin and Adderall, while others are given drugs to deal with depression and anxiety, like Prozac and Zoloft.[67]

These drugs are more familiar to a general population in North America and Western Europe. Their use is controversial and sometimes stigmatized, just as it is in the neurotypical population. This can make an autistic person feel even more like they are broken and in need of fixing, even if the drugs prescribed are necessary.

There has also been an extra challenge related to coexisting diagnoses. Doctors sometimes do not know whether to treat the symptoms related to autism or the coexisting conditions. Because certain drugs are approved for autism in children, some doctors may see that as generalizable to adults.[68] While this *can* work, sometimes doctors are more reluctant to prescribe medication at all if they do not feel they have the experience necessary to do so responsibly. This means many autistic adults can go without medications that could help them.[69]

This is related to the problem of public perception, including by physicians. If even a doctor, who is supposed to know about autism, does not understand it well enough to properly prescribe medications, how confident can an autistic person be about how the rest of the world is supposed to see them?

Issues related to this misperception informs the second kind of drug use, one that is related to illegal or at least recreational kinds of drugs. Here, there are some notable trends. Prevalence rates of drug use among autistic people are in dispute, but a 2021 study in *The Lancet* found that autistic people were less likely than the general population to use drugs.[70] However, it also found they were more likely to use drugs to "manage mental health symptoms."[71] In other words, it seems more probable that autistic people are less likely to use illegal drugs recreationally, but they may take them to control issues with conditions like anxiety and depression if they see this as preferable to living with these conditions.

Though more research is needed, evidence suggests that autistic women use more recreational drugs than men, which is possibly related to them having more suicide attempts and a lower quality of life overall.[72] This may also be related to self-soothing types of behaviour.

These findings relate to an observation about autistic people in general that comes from researchers including Susan Lowinger, which may be one of the most important traits to consider when an autistic person uses recreational drugs: "searching for excitement and novelty are not prominent traits of those with ASD, whereas rigidity and adherence to laws and rules, even in the face of social pressure, absolutely are."[73]

Drug use, especially of a recreational kind, can also be linked to one of the ultimate negative consequences in life — the legal system. This is where autistic people, drug users or not, can find themselves in real trouble.

## Criminality

Mark Haddon's bestselling 2003 book, *The Curious Incident of the Dog in the Night-Time*, begins with British autistic protagonist Christopher Boone, age fifteen, finding a dead dog in his neighbour's front yard. He is fond of the dog, and its death, which he rightly suspects was murder, disturbs him greatly.

When the police see Christopher clutching the dead dog out of despair and sadness, he is mistaken to be the killer. His behaviour included being overwhelmed and not talking to the police, to putting his hands on the one who touched him, and to being overly honest in the police station when his father arrives.

Eventually, the police realize Christopher could not have killed the dog, and his father picks him up later that night. This fictional encounter illustrates what kinds of real problems autistic people can face when they encounter the police, and how autistic people perceive themselves when others see them as criminals.

This example takes a couple of big lessons from real life. The data has been clear about criminality in autism for a long time: like Christopher, *autistic people in general are no more likely to commit violent crimes than the general population.*[74] They are more likely to be victims than perpetrators of crimes.[75]

There are some distinctions about whether autistic people may be more likely to cause certain kinds of crimes, or whether they are more likely to encounter a police officer.[76] But the data is clear that, overall, they are not more likely to be criminals than other people.

Despite this well-known fact, autistic people, like Christopher, can make others suspicious in criminal matters. According to some studies, evidence suggests that, in police interviews, autistic people are more likely to be believed to be criminals than neurotypicals. This is largely because their unconventional social manner sometimes exhibits what others think of as tells that are not, in fact, reflecting deception. This can include not giving eye contact, freezing during a question because of nerves, or showing signs of distress that are more likely due to presence of trouble rather than guilt.[77]

This perception of being bad, even if it is not reflecting reality, can impact how autistic people see themselves. Whether it is doing something that makes them look guilty of a crime, or whether they say something rude at a professional occasion, others seeing them as bad can be internalized by the time they are adults.[78] Like other people in similar scenarios, sometimes they can even learn to play the part.

Will Attwood, Tony Attwood's son, is an autistic man who committed an armed robbery related to a drug addiction. This crime earned him a three-year prison sentence in Australia, during which he was diagnosed with Asperger's syndrome.[79]

He has since written a book about autism and the criminal justice system called *Asperger's Syndrome and Jail* in which he gives advice to autistic people who end up in the legal system. The first part of his book contains essential advice: stay out of prison to begin with. For most autistic people, like most others, this is accomplished. But if an autistic person does end up in prison, they experience special issues there.

Attwood says that the prison he was in was not quite the violent "don't drop the soap" experience that is sometimes portrayed. It is nevertheless a tense place where following social rules and conventions can make meaningful differences in a person's prison experience. Even prisoners who may be less intelligent from an IQ sense can do better in prison if they know the unspoken rules of what to do and not to do.[80]

Being autistic in a world where others might laugh or be offended at their traits can be emotionally challenging. Being autistic in a world where physical and mental toughness, including high social awareness, is the key variable to get through everyday life can be outright dangerous. For this reason, prisons have special needs units that are designed to help protect people who are from more perilous circumstances. These units generally offer a "less dangerous and more relaxed atmosphere," according to Attwood.[81] However, an inmate can not just ask to be put in this unit; usually staff will place a patient there after exhausting every other avenue. It is also not as if these units do not have their own difficulties; they are considered the "end of the road," to use Attwood's words (places where only the most difficult prisoners go).[82]

The quality of data, especially comparing autistic to non-autistic prisoners, still lacks evidence showing just how the criminal justice system is different for autistic people.[83] If someone like Attwood is an indication, it does have some special considerations, but it is a survivable experience.

Another question is what happens when autistic people get out of prison. Since they often have a difficult time getting jobs anyway, a criminal record can be especially detrimental to their ability to lead a normal life.

Will Attwood, for instance, lived with his parents well into his thirties, battling the drug addiction he has faced since his teen years, when he started taking drugs to calm anxiety that he now attributes to being autistic.[84] As drug use and crime can sometimes coincide, helping to lower the causes of drug use in autistic people would help prevent them from ending up in the criminal justice system in the first place. Autistic people do not commit crimes because of drug use. Although the range of crimes autistic people commit varies as much as in the neurotypical population, their motives can differ.

For example, stalking can be as much a matter of lacking social understanding as it is about intimidation, such as a general lack of understanding for personal space. Sexual crimes, while they can be motivated by something nefarious, can be committed out of sheer ignorance or rigidity in interpreting social rules. An autistic person might say something that sounds threatening to most people, but it is really their way of expressing frustration. As described earlier in Darius McCollum's case, it can serve a need.

In many respects, the criminality of autistic people sums up the traits and issues covered throughout this book and shows the worst of what can happen when autistic people are neglected and misunderstood. As adults, they can do negative things to themselves and others, just as people who go through adverse experiences in general are more likely to do.

## Conclusion

It is arguable, though highly plausible, that problems of self-perception are at the root of many of the most endemic and tragic issues in the autistic community. What kills autistic adults and cripples their lives primarily have to do with how they view themselves. Problems like drug use and criminality, and issues with sexuality come from low self-esteem, which can result from low expectations from others and trauma.

In a sense, the problems of self-understanding do also come from other causes. If the people who conduct research about autistic people do not care enough to know about what they are studying, the people responsible for providing quality services cannot fully do their job.

If the public does not get an accurate picture or good information about who autistic people are, they are more inclined to discriminate. When the entire society does not adequately care about them, that leaves autistic adults with poor self-perception. If no one else thinks they matter, they won't think they matter either. This is tragic.

Throughout the book, there are examples of autistic people having unique challenges, but they also have many gifts. These can be intellectual gifts that a happy and self-caring person can use to feed themselves and their families, and they can be unique extremes of honesty, goodness, and generosity they can provide to others. Society as a whole would do better by recognizing these qualities. If everyone else does, it is more likely that autistic people will as well.

However, like all people, autistic adults must also find meaning and strength within themselves. All people suffer, and all people have challenges. There is a lot the broader society can do; autistic people must do the rest. Just like everyone else, they must find their own interests and identities. This comes through building up enough self-confidence and competence to do what is needed to survive to the best of their ability.

This looks different for diverse autistic people. For someone with a higher-than-average IQ and a fierce interest in medicine, this can mean being happy in a medical career. For another with an intellectual disability and a big heart, this can be working as a department store greeter who makes the people who walk in happier.

As difficult as society can sometimes make things for autistic people, and a lot of work must still be done to fix these problems, it is easier than ever for them to get into school, to find jobs, and to secure accommodations. Anyone who forms an opinion of themselves based on other people's perceptions is doing themselves a disservice in the long run.

The road is hard, likely harder than for others, but ultimately not travelling it is harder on their body, their mind, and their soul.

# CONCLUSION

LIFE HAS SIMULTANEOUSLY BECOME MUCH MORE complicated and meaningful since I was that little kid saying numbers on the soccer field. I have seen and experienced a lot since then, some of which has harshly woken me up in ways I think many neurotypicals don't go through.

When your brain works in a way that makes you feel like an alien to other people, whether it is through your senses, your social expectations, or the ways you soothe yourself, it can be every bit as othering to the rest of society as any other way a person could be seen as not fully "one of us." This means that autistic adults see the world as perpetual outsiders. While neurotypicals must also learn about the world when growing up, they more often learn with the support and understanding of others. This can be through shared experiences with peers or through understanding elders.

While autistic people can get crucial support throughout their lives, these lessons are more often learned as a surprise and even an affront to their basic assumptions. This means they constantly see the world in ways that are different — some that are useful and others that are deeply confusing and even painful.

By the time autistic people are adults, they find a lot of methods to deal with this. Some paths, like delving into a personal interest that helps others, are generally healthier. Other paths, like isolation and drug use, are high risk and can easily end in disaster, including even premature death. Many autistic people are somewhere in between these two places.

One lesson I've learned is that a person's quality of life is ultimately reflected in how they feel about themselves even more than how others view them. I believe this is one of the most important lessons anyone can learn, especially autistic people.

Self-esteem should be earned by what a person does, as a person should not have an inflated view of their own abilities. But a person's essential self-worth also should not be dependent on what others think of them, especially when conventional standards are often not sufficient to apply to their lives.

While this balance should be kept in mind for anyone, for autistic people this also sets up a more difficult standard. Because of the inherent limitations they will always have, they will likely never seem fully neurotypical. But the world often compares autistic people to neurotypical standards, which means they are often seen to fall short.

This is a harsher standard than most people are held to, and one that can even be impossible to live up to. *It is important to recognize an autistic person and understand when an autistic person is trying their best.* People should also recognize an autistic person's virtues that exist not despite autism but because of autism.

However, there's also a flip side to this difficulty. In my experience, most autistic people say they would not be neurotypical if they had the choice. Traits that can seem strange to others mean a lot and are beneficial for an autistic person, which complicate how they must go through life. Autism's difficulties mean that they often must figure out which parts of themselves they must protect and which they should work to let go so they can mature.

This is especially crucial as an adolescent and into adulthood, as people are discovering their identity. All people must ask themselves questions like this, but for autistic people who can be bullied and ostracized for traits that harm no one, it can sometimes be an especially confusing and difficult process. "The world tells me this is wrong, but I know it's not wrong. Who should I believe?"

All people deal with this to some degree, but as with many things about being autistic, this is taken to the extreme. What neurotypical people often do not realize is that while autistic people can be stubborn, bitter, frustrating, and needlessly clueless of others' feelings, they can also be kind, sincere, gifted, and untethered to conventions that really are outdated or needless. This is true of all autistic people, regardless of the obviousness of their autism to outsiders.

It's getting to know both sides of autistic people that many neurotypicals sadly may not have the patience for. I hope that this book will have provoked thoughts that inform and foster this patience.

Autistic people, adults especially, also have more needs beyond the patience of their peers. Many autistic adults face material difficulties. While there has been progress in treating autistic people in beneficial ways, there is still a long way to go. The question is how to do it, and there is a lot of disagreement and many limitations on this.

Despite the differences between the autism and autistic communities, and the different ways they see the issues surrounding autism, there are some goals for helping autistic adults that almost everyone would agree on that help with these material differences:

- Find more ways and resources to identify and diagnose more autistic people, especially among groups like women, ethnic minorities, and people of different sex and gender orientations
- Find ways to shorten the waiting lists for residential care, which allows autistic residents to be full members of the community, and improve quality of services in these care homes
- Get rid of the "marriage penalty"
- Find ways to shorten the waiting lists for access to therapy
- Find ways to encourage mutual understanding between autistic and neurotypical people, especially in cases where they are more likely to see each other as strangers at first

My hope is that these goals can be a starting point for a united autism rights movement without divisions between active parents and active autistic adults because most organizations benefit from being united.

After hearing many points of view and having a lifetime of being autistic, I'm convinced that dialogue between people is more productive than antagonizing others, which happens too often in this community.

I understand why this divide exists. Unlike most medical concerns, autism is more complex, often more philosophically charged, and full of values clashes, not just differences on how to attain agreed goals. The science around autism, especially in adults, can be vague, which only makes having agreed goals even more confusing.

Given where both groups are at right now, I don't expect a reconciliation to happen any time soon. The world of autism will likely remain a divided and combative realm. However, I don't think it needs to be, nor is it in the best interest of autistic people for it to be that way. Both communities can learn important things from each other.

Ultimately, on a social level, I think autistic adults and neurotypicals need to meet each other halfway. The experiences and personalities of autistic adults are as real as anyone else's. If autism is best understood as a culture, the rest of society needs to understand it the same way they understand different cultures and sexual orientations.

Autistic people also need to understand how the rest of the world thinks and make certain accommodations that are possible without fundamentally changing who they are. Not asking this of an autistic person is a bit like not asking a paraplegic to go through rehab and learn how to use a wheelchair.

Generally, autistic people, including many in the autistic community, agree with this at some level. As Ari Ne'eman, the founder of the Autism Self-Advocacy Network, once told an ABC interviewer in 2008, "anti-cure doesn't mean anti-progress."[1] Even large parts of the self-advocacy movement, focused on the happiness of autistic people, understand that certain ways of learning the ways of the world will increase their overall happiness in the end.

While it is a greater challenge for autistic people to learn skills in life, they are not asked to do something that all people are not fundamentally asked to do. That is, they are asked to learn and grow from training and experience. The test for everyone should be: do you try?

This is on an individual level. Some people may read this book looking for big solutions to the problems it addressed. They may be disappointed that I largely do not provide them.

I do not know how to reform government and private services. I do not know every possible way to reasonably accommodate autistic people. I do not know how to reform residential care to make it more accessible for autistic adults, and I do not know how to make the workplace accessible for every autistic adult who can work.

Any progress that is likely to be made on these fronts is going to be slow. It takes a long time for the research literature to emerge with solid data and findings even on minor issues relating to autistic adults. Once those are evident, forming services and health care that address the needs of autistic people takes even longer.

This may not be satisfying for many autistic adults, who have daily struggles that in an ideal world would be solved now. Unfortunately, the world is where it is, and the best anyone can do is to make it slightly better today than it was yesterday.

If there *is* a big take-away a reader should come away with and apply to their lives, it is that their attitude towards autistic adults is just as key as any other factor.

What causes autistic people more pain than perhaps anything else in their experience is the attitudes of other people towards their differences. Acceptance and understanding go a long way.

Although this can be taught in an education system, it is most effectively taught through each person's own experience. Tony Attwood once said something that I feel perfectly sums up what I would say to neurotypical people who may have an autistic person in their lives:

> I think people with autism are heroes. I think if you could be autistic for a day, you would completely change your attitude. They cope, they strive to cope, in a world of social zealots, and if I was going to change one thing, it would be appreciation of the challenges the person faces, and not to assume that they're stupid, or to assume that they're bad or naughty. A lot of the things that they do are just coping mechanisms with life. If I was going to change anything in life, it would be attitude towards such individuals. And sometimes attitude, dare I say this, is free.[2]

I believe many autistic people would echo this sentiment. Being understood and treated with courtesy makes as much difference as climbing the waiting list for a service. This is also one area where the autism and autistic communities should agree.

If the goal of the autism community is to help autistic people integrate into wider society, that will be more likely if they feel that wider society respects them to begin with. If the goal of the autistic community is to have autistic people more accepted for who they are, improving attitudes goes a long way towards this goal.

Autistic adults may seem a little strange on first impression, but they are fundamentally like anyone else you know. When service providers, governments, researchers, and laypeople act like this is true, the autistic people in this remarkable community lead happier lives.

# NOTES

## Introduction

1. I don't speak Bahasa Indonesian at all today. When I was four, we went to live in the United States and Canada for the rest of my childhood.

## Chapter 1: A History and Overview of Autism

1. *Screening and Diagnosis of Autism Spectrum Disorder*, March 31, 2022. Retrieved May 9, 2022, from www.cdc.gov/ncbddd/autism/screening.html

2. Attwood, T., *The Complete Guide to Asperger's Syndrome*, 2nd ed., Jessica Kingsley, 2015, 72–74.

3. Brian, J.A., L. Zwaigenbaum, and A. Ip, "Standards of Diagnostic Assessment for Autism Spectrum Disorder," October 24, 2019. Retrieved May 9, 2022, from https://cps.ca/documents/position/asd-diagnostic-assessment

4. Centers for Disease Control and Prevention, *Diagnostic Criteria for 299.00 Autism Spectrum Disorder,* April 6, 2022. Retrieved May 11, 2022, from www.cdc.gov/ncbddd/autism/hcp-dsm.html

5. Carpenter, L., "DSM-5 Autism Spectrum Disorder: Guidelines and Criteria Exemplars," February 2013. Retrieved May 11, 2022, from https://depts.washington.edu

6. Ibid.

7. Lowry, L., "'He Was Talking and Then He Just Stopped': A Look at Regression in Autism," The Hanen Centre, n.d. Retrieved May 11, 2022, from www.hanen.org

8. Flannery K.A., and R. Wisner-Carlson, "Autism and Education," *Child Adolescent Psychiatric Clinics of North America*, 29(2), 2020, 319–43.

9. Wing, L., *The Autism Spectrum: A Guide for Parents and Professionals*, Constable and Robinson, 2002, 22–23.

10. Grandin, T., "Thinking the Way Animals Do: Unique Insights from a Person with Singular Understanding," *Western Horseman*, November 1997, 140–45.

11. Howlin, P., *Autism and Asperger Syndrome: Preparing for Adulthood*, 2nd ed., Routledge Taylor and Francis Group, 2004, 320.

12. Generation Next, *Could It Be Asperger's?* Video, January 25, 2015, www.youtube.com/watch?v=LuZFThlOiJI

13. Attwood, *The Complete Guide to Asperger's Syndrome*, 113–14.

14. Ibid., 103–04.

15. Silberman, S., *NeuroTribes: The Legacy of Autism and the Future of Neurodiversity*, Avery Publishing, 2015, 19–44; Donvan, J and C. Zucker, *In a Different Key: The Story of Autism*, Broadway Books, 2016, 553.

16. Evans, B., "How Autism Became Autism: The Radical Transformation of a Central Concept of Child Development in Britain," *History of the Human Sciences*, 26(3), 2013, 3–31; Posar, A., and P. Visconti., "Tribute to Grunya Efimovna Sukhareva, the Woman Who First Described Infantile Autism," *Journal of Pediatric Neurosciences*, 12(3), 2017, 300–01.

17. Kanner, L., "Autistic Disturbances of Affective Contact," *Nervous Child, 2*, 1943, 217–50.

18. Arnold, C., "Autism's Race Problem," *Pacific Standard*, June 14, 2017.

19. "Donald Triplett, 'Case 1' in the Study of Autism, Dies at 89," Obituaries, *New York Times*, June 18, 2023. Retrieved August 9, 2023, from https://www.nytimes.com/2023/06/18/obituaries/donald-triplett-dead.html

20. Silberman, *NeuroTribes*, 93.

21. Reynolds, C.R., K.J. Vannest, and E. Fletcher-Janzen, eds., *Encyclopedia of Special Education Volume 1: A Reference for the Education of Children, Adolescents, and Adults Disabilities and Other Individuals*, Wiley, 2014.

22. Science Direct, *Autistic Psychopathy*. Retrieved May 11, 2022, from sciencedirect.com.

23. Silberman, *NeuroTribes*, 93.

24. Donvan and Zucker, *In a Different Key*, 319.

25. Silberman, *NeuroTribes*,167–69.

26. Kanner, "Autistic Disturbances," 217–50.

27. Donvan and Zucker, *In a Different Key*, 322.

28. Stagslad, K., "Asperger, the Nazis and the Children: The History of the Birth of a Diagnosis," Tidsskriftet, May 16, 2019. Retrieved May 14, 2022, from https://tidsskriftet.no

29. Donvan and Zucker, *In a Different Key*, 318.

30. Ibid., 338.

31. Czech, H., "Hans Asperger, National Socialism, and 'Race Hygiene' in Nazi-era Vienna," *Molecular Autism*, 9, 2018, 1–43.

32. National Academies of Sciences, Engineering, and Medicine, "Prevalence of Autism Spectrum Disorder," in *Mental Disorders and Disabilities among Low-Income Children*, eds. T.F. Boat and J.T. Wu, The National Academies Press, 2015, https://www.ncbi.nlm.nih.gov/books/NBK332882/.

33. Grandin, T., *Emergence: Labelled Autistic*, Warner Books, 1986, 2005, 24.

34. Masi, G., and F. Liboni, "Management of Schizophrenia in Children and Adolescents," *Drugs*, 71, 2011, 179–208.

35. Donvan and Zucker, *In a Different Key*, 148.

36. Silberman, *NeuroTribes*, 279.

37. Dibden, E., "The Heartbreaking True Story of the Queen's Cousins, Nerissa and Katherine Bowes-Lyon," *Harper's Bazaar*, November 21, 2020.

38. Senate of Canada Report, Standing Senate Committee on Social Affairs, Science and Technology, "Mental Health Service Delivery and Addiction Treatment in Canada: An Historical Perspective," in *Mental Health, Mental Illness, and Addiction: Overview of Policies and Programs in Canada*, November 2004.

39. Natoli, A.P., "The DSM's Reconnection to Psychoanalytic Theory Through the Alternative Model for Personality Disorders," *Journal of the American Psychoanalytic Association*, 67(6), 2019, 1023–45.

40. Donvan and Zucker, *In a Different Key*, 89–90.

41. Grossman, R., "Genius or Fraud? Bettelheim's Biographers Can't Seem to Decide," *Chicago Tribune*, January 23, 1997.

42. Nuwar, R., "Autism's History Holds Lessons for Today's Researchers," *Spectrum*, March 14, 2016. Retrieved November 10, 2022, from www.spectrumnews.org.

43. Rimland, B., *Infantile Autism: The Syndrome and Its Implications for a Neural Theory of Behavior*, Jessica Kingsley, 2015, 46.

44. Lord, C., et al., "Autism Spectrum Disorder," *Nature Reviews Disease Primers*, 6(5), 2020, 5.

45. Kanner, L., "Follow-up Study of Eleven Autistic Children Originally Reported in 1943," *Focus on Autistic Behaviour, 7(5)*, 1992, 1–11.

46. Volkmar, F.R., B. Reichow, and J.C. McPartland, *Adolescents and Adults with Autism Spectrum Disorders*, Springer Science + Business Media, 2014, 29.

47. *What Is TEACCH?* Retrieved May 14, 2022, from www.autismspeaks.org/teacch-0

48. Smith, T., and S.O. Eikeseth, "Ivar Lovaas: Pioneer of Applied Behavior Analysis and Intervention for Children with Autism," *Journal of Autism and Developmental Disorders*, 41, 2011, 375–78.

49. Donvan and Zucker, *In a Different Key*, 241–46.

50. Yu, Q., E. Li, L. Li, and W. Liang, "Efficacy of Interventions Based on Applied Behavior Analysis for Autism Spectrum Disorder: A Meta-Analysis," *Psychiatry Investigation*, 17(5), 2020, 432–43.

51. Ronald, A., and R. Plomin, "1977 Paper on the First Autism Twin Study," *Spectrum*, March 19, 2008. Retrieved November 10, 2022, from www.spectrumnews.com

52. Baron-Cohen, S. and A. Klin, "What's So Special About Asperger's Syndrome?" *Brain and Cognition*, 61, 2006, 1–4.

53. Greener, M., "DSM-5: Rewriting the 'Bible,'" *Progress in Neurology and Psychiatry*, 2013, 24–6.

54. Schopler, E., "Introduction," in E. Schopler and G.B. Mesibov, eds., *Autism in Adolescents and Adults, Current Issues in Autism*, Springer Science + Business Media, 1983, 3-10.

55. Happé, F., and S. Baron-Cohen, "Remembering Lorna Wing (1928–2014)," *Spectrum*, July 15, 2014. Retrieved November 10, 2022, from www.spectrumnews.com

56. Donvan and Zucker, *In a Different Key*, 409–14.

57. Ottawa-Carleton Association for Persons with Developmental Disabilities, *Silver Spring Farm*. Retrieved November 19, 2022, from www.ocapdd.on.ca

58. Giddan, N.S., and J. Jane, eds., *Autistic Adults at Bittersweet Farms*, Routledge, 1991, 17.

59. Ibid., 65–6.

60. Torquati, B., et al., "Social Farming and Work Inclusion Initiatives for Adults

with Autism Spectrum Disorders: A Pilot Study," *NJAS: Wageningen Journal of Life Sciences, 88,* 2019, 10–20; *Bittersweet Farms*, n.d. Retrieved November 19, 2022, from www.bittersweetfarms.org; Artz, B., and D.B. Davis, "Green Care: A Review of the Benefits and Potential of Animal-Assisted Care Farming Globally and in Rural America," *Animals*, 7(4), 2017, 31.

61. *A History of the Individuals with Disabilities Education Act*, March 18, 2022. Retrieved May 11, 2022, from https://sites.ed.gov/idea/IDEA-History

62. Rimand, B., in T. Grandin, *Emergence: Labeled Autistic*, Warner, 1986, 2005, 3.

63. Pripas-Kapit, S., "Historicizing Jim Sinclair's 'Don't Mourn for Us': A Cultural and Intellectual History of Neurodiversity's First Manifesto," in *Autistic Community and the Neurodiversity Movement*, S. Kapp, ed., Palgrave Macmillan, 2020, 23-39.

64. Sinclair, J., "Don't Mourn for Us," *Autonomy: The Critical Journal of Interdisciplinary Autism Studies,* 1(1), 2012, 1–4.

65. Howlin, "Introduction," in *Autism and Asperger Syndrome*, 1.

66. Silberman, S., "The Geek Syndrome," Wired.com, December 1, 2001.

67. "2015 The Baillie Gifford Prize for Non-Fiction," n.d. www.thebailliegifford-prize.co.uk/year-by-year/2015

68. *Search: autism adults.* Retrieved November 10, 2022, from https://pubmed.ncbi.nlm.nih.gov

69. Donvan and Zucker, *In a Different Key*, 395–6.

70. *Autism Speaks, Autism Speaks and Cure Autism Now Complete Merger: Combined Operations of Leading Autism Organizations Will Lead to Enhanced Research, Treatment and Advocacy Programs,* February 5, 2007. Retrieved November 10, 2022, from https://www.autismspeaks.org/about-agre

71. Donvan and Zucker, *In a Different Key*, 465.

72. Gernsbacher, M.A., et al., "Do Puzzle Pieces and Autism Puzzle Piece Logos Evoke Negative Associations?" *Autism: The International Journal of Research and Practice*, 22(2), 2018, 118–25.

73. ASAN, *Before You Donate to Autism Speaks, Consider the Facts.* Retrieved November 10, 2022, from https://autisticadvocacy.org

74. Robison, J.E., "My Time with Autism Speaks," in *Autistic Community and the Neurodiversity Movement*, S. Kapp, ed., Palgrave Macmillan, 2020.

75. Luterman, S., "The Biggest Autism Advocacy Group Is Still Failing Too Many Autistic People," *Washington Post,* February 14, 2020.

76. Autism Speaks, *Questions and Answers: Why Did Autism Speaks Remove 'Cure' from Its Mission and Research?* Retrieved November 10, 2022, from www.autismspeaks.org

77. Rao, T.S., and C. Andrade, "The MMR Vaccine and Autism: Sensation, Refutation, Retraction, and Fraud," *Indian Journal of Psychiatry*, 53(2), 2011, 95–6.

78. Carey, B., "Bernard Rimland, 78, Scientist Who Revised View of Autism, Dies," *New York Times,* November 28, 2006.

79. U.S. House Government Reform Committee, *Vaccines and the Autism Epidemic: Reviewing the Federal Government's Track Record and Charting a Course for the Future,*

December 10, 2002. Retrieved May 13, 2022, from www.congress.gov

80. Meikle, J., and S. Bosely, "MMR Row Doctor Andrew Wakefield Struck Off Register," *The Guardian,* May 24, 2010.

81. Bever, L., "Autism Speaks, Leading Autism Advocate, Urges Vaccination," *Washington Post,* February 9, 2015.

82. Reed, G.M., et al., "Innovations and Changes in the ICD-11 Classification of Mental, Behavioural and Developmental Disorders," *World Psychiatry*, 18(1), February 2019, 3–19.

83. Attwood, *The Complete Guide to Asperger's Syndrome*, 57.

84. Zeldovich, L., "Why the Definition of Autism Needs to Be Refined," *Spectrum,* May 18, 2018. Retrieved November 10, 2022, from www.spectrumnews.org

85. Volkmar, Reichow, and McPartland, *Adolescents and Adults with Autism Spectrum Disorders*, 1.

86. Ibid.

## Chapter 2: Autistic Adults Today

1. Centers for Disease Control and Prevention, *Data & Statistics on Autism Spectrum Disorder*. Retrieved November 10, 2022, from www.cdc.gov/ncbddd/autism/data.html

2. Gates, G.J., "How Many People Are Lesbian, Gay, Bisexual, and Transgender?" UCLA School of Law, Williams Institute, April 2011. Retrieved August 9, 2023, from https://williamsinstitute.law.ucla.edu; Brandeis, *American Jewish Population Project,* revised May 18, 2021. Retrieved August 9, 2023, from https://ajpp.brandeis.edu; Mohamed, B., "New Estimates Show U.S. Muslim Population Continues to Grow," Pew Research Center, January 3, 2018. Retrieved May 13, 2022, from https://www.pewresearch.org

3. Centers for Disease Control and Prevention, *Data & Statistics on Autism Spectrum Disorder*, March 2, 2022. Retrieved May 14, 2022, from www.cdc.gov/ncbddd/autism/data.html; Autism and Developmental Disabilities Monitoring Network Surveillance Year 2000 Principal Investigators, Centers for Disease Control and Prevention, "Prevalence of Autism Spectrum Disorders Autism and Developmental Disabilities Monitoring Network, Six Sites, United States, 2000," *MMWR Surveillance Summaries*, 56(1), February 9, 2007, 1–11.

4. Peart, K.N., "Prevalence of Autism in South Korea Estimated at 1 in 38 Children," *YaleNews*, May 9, 2011. Retrieved May 13, 2022, from https://news.yale.edu

5. Burgha, T., "Epidemiology of Autism Spectrum Disorders in Adults in the Community in England," *Archives of General Psychiatry*, 68(5), 2011, 459–65.

6. Hoover, D.W., and J. Kaufman, "Adverse Childhood Experiences in Children with Autism Spectrum Disorder," *Current Opinion in Psychiatry*, 31(2), 2018, 128–32.

7. Kerns, C.M., C.J. Newschaffer, S. Berkowitz, and B.K. Lee, "Brief Report: Examining the Association of Autism and Adverse Childhood Experiences in the National Survey of Children's Health: The Important Role of Income and Co-occurring Mental Health Conditions," *Journal of Autism and Developmental Disorders*, 47(7), 2017, 2275–81.

8. DeAngelis, T., "Losing an Autism Diagnosis," *American Psychological Association*, 50(4), 2019, 22.

9. Gerdts, J., and R. Bernier, "The Broader Autism Phenotype and Its Implications on the Etiology and Treatment of Autism Spectrum Disorders," *Autism Research and Treatment*, 2011, article no. 545901; Sasson, N.J., et al., "Autism and the Broad Autism Phenotype: Familial Patterns and Intergenerational Transmission," *Journal of Neurodevelopmental Disorders*, 5(11), 2013.

10. Rubenstein, E., and D. Chawla, "Broader Autism Phenotype in Parents of Children with Autism: A Systematic Review of Percentage Estimates," *Journal of Child and Family Studies*, 27(6), 2018, 1705–20.

11. Kanner, L., "Autistic Disturbances of Affective Contact, *Nervous Child, 2,* 1943, 217–250. Kanner wrote in this original paper of how some of the people he studied have "beautiful" faces.

12. Coon, H., in *Autism Spectrum Disorder in Mid and Later Life,* S.D. Wright, ed., Jessica Kingsley, 2015, 54.

13. Lockwood Estrin, G., et al., "Barriers to Autism Spectrum Disorder Diagnosis for Young Women and Girls: A Systematic Review," *Review Journal of Autism and Developmental Disorders*, 8, 2021, 454–70. This source particularly looks at this issue with autistic women, but it can happen with autistic men as well.

14. Howlin, P., *Autism and Asperger Syndrome: Preparing for Adulthood*, 2nd ed., Routledge Taylor and Francis Group, 2004, 3.

15. Asperger, H., "'Autistic Psychopathy' in Childhood," in *Autism and Asperger Syndrome*, U. Frith, ed., Cambridge University Press, 1991, 44.

16. Budryk, Z., "More Celebrities Are Coming Out as Autistic: That Makes a Huge Difference," *Washington Post*, September 4, 2021; "Elon Musk Reveals He Has Asperger's on Saturday Night Live," *BBC News,* May 9, 2021.

17. Stoddart, K., L. Burke, and R. King., *Asperger Syndrome in Adulthood: A Comprehensive Guide for Clinicians*, W.W. Norton, 2012, 197.

## Chapter 3: Social Communication

1. Nguyen, W., et al., "How I See and Feel About Myself: Domain-Specific Self-Concept and Self-Esteem in Autistic Adults," *Frontiers in Psychology*, 2020.

2. Williams, G. L., Wharton, T., and Jagoe, C., "Mutual (Mis)understanding: Reframing Autistic Pragmatic 'Impairments' Using Relevance Theory," *Frontiers in Psychology*, 12, 2021; Whelan, C., "Infodumping: Autistic Love Language," *Autistic Rights* (blog), July 16, 2020. Retrieved November 10, 2022, from https://autisticrights.net.

3. Howlin, P., *Autism and Asperger Syndrome: Preparing for Adulthood*, 2nd ed., Routledge Taylor and Francis Group, 2004, 176.

4. Donvan and Zucker, *In a Different Key*, 537.

5. Kalandadze, T., et al., "Metaphor Comprehension in Individuals with Autism

Spectrum Disorder: Core Language Skills Matter," *Journal of Autism Developmental Disorders*, 52, 2022, 316–26.

6. Izuma, K., et al., "Insensitivity to Social Reputation in Autism," *Proceedings of the National Academy of Sciences*, 108(42), 2011.

7. Attwood, T., *The Complete Guide to Asperger's Syndrome*, 2nd ed., Jessica Kingsley Publishers, 2015, 70.

8. Kennedy, D.P., and R. Adolphs, "Violations of Personal Space by Individuals with Autism Spectrum Disorder," *PLOS ONE*, 9(8), 2014, 1–10.

9. Barzeva, S.A., W.H.J. Meeus, and A.J. Oldehinkel, "Social Withdrawal in Adolescence and Early Adulthood: Measurement Issues, Normative Development, and Distinct Trajectories," *Journal of Abnormal Child Psychology*, 47, 2019, 865–79.

10. Asperger, H., "'Autistic Psychopathy' in Childhood," in *Autism and Asperger Syndrome*, U. Frith, ed., Cambridge University Press, 1991, 42.

11. Woodbury-Smith, M.R., and F.R. Volkmar, "Asperger Syndrome," *European Child & Adolescent Psychiatry*, 18(1), 2008, 2–11.

12. Sohn, E., "How Abuse Mars the Lives of Autistic People," *Spectrum*, February 5, 2020. Retrieved November 10, 2022, from www.spectrumnews.org

13. Huang, A.X., et al., "Understanding the Self in Individuals with Autism Spectrum Disorders (ASD): A Review of Literature," *Frontiers in Psychology*, 8, 2017, 1422.

14. Stoddart, K., L. Burke, and R. King., *Asperger Syndrome in Adulthood: A Comprehensive Guide for Clinicians*, W.W. Norton, 2012, 102.

15. Person requested anonymity.

16. Attwood, *The Complete Guide to Asperger's Syndrome*, 59–60.

17. Ibid.

18. Ibid., 31–2.

19. Ibid., xx.

20. Ibid., 70.

21. Ibid.

22. Ibid.

23. Howlin, *Autism and Asperger Syndrome*, 140–1.

24. Fujino, J., et al., "Need for Closure and Cognitive Flexibility in Individuals with Autism Spectrum Disorder: A Preliminary Study," *Psychiatry Research*, 271, 2019, 247–52.

25. Attwood, *The Complete Guide to Asperger's Syndrome*, 35–40.

26. Generation Next, *Could It Be Asperger's?* Video, January 25, 2015, www.youtube.com/watch?v=LuZFThlOiJI

27. Wimmer, H., and J. Perner, "Beliefs about Beliefs: Representation and Constraining Function of Wrong Beliefs in Young Children's Understanding of Deception," *Cognition*, 13(1), 1983,103–28.

28. Leslie, A.M., and U. Frith, "Autistic Children's Understanding of Seeing, Knowing and Believing," *British Journal of Developmental Psychology*, 6(4), 1988, 315–24.

29. Baron-Cohen, S., A.M. Leslie, and U. Frith, "Does the Autistic Child Have a 'Theory of Mind'?" *Cognition*, 21(1), 1985, 37–46.

30. Hynes, C.A., A.A. Baird, and S.T. Grafton, "Differential Role of the Orbital Frontal Lobe in Emotional Versus Cognitive Perspective-Taking," *Neuropsychologia*, 44(3), 2006, 374–83.

31. Baron-Cohen, S., *The Pattern Seekers: How Autism Drives Human Invention*, Basic Books, 2020, 79.

32. Senju, A., "Spontaneous Theory of Mind and Its Absence in Autism Spectrum Disorders," *The Neuroscientist*, 18(2), 2012, 108–13.

33. Beaudoin, C., et al., "Systematic Review and Inventory of Theory of Mind Measures for Young Children," *Frontiers in Psychology*, 10, 2020, https://www.frontiersin.org/articles/10.3389/fpsyg.2019.02905/full

34. Bloom, P., and T.P. German, "Two Reasons to Abandon the False Belief Task as a Test of Theory of Mind," *Cognition*, 77, 2000, B25–31.

35. Milton, D., "On the Ontological Status of Autism: The 'Double Empathy Problem,'" *Disability & Society*, 27(6), 2012, 883–87.

36. Ibid.

37. I must give credit here to the National Autistic Society in England for their excellent summary of the double empathy problem, where I was introduced to these papers. That summary can be found here: Milton, D., "The Double Empathy Problem," National Autistic Society, March 2, 2018. Retrieved November 10, 2022, from www.autism.org.uk

38. Heasman, B., and A. Gillespie, "Perspective-taking Is Two-sided: Misunderstandings Between People with Asperger's Syndrome and Their Family Members," *Autism: The International Journal of Research and Practice*, 22(6), 2018, 740–50.

39. Casartelli, L., et al., "Neurotypical Individuals Fail to Understand Action Vitality Form in Children with Autism Spectrum Disorder," *Proceedings of the National Academy of Sciences*, 117(44), 2020.

40. Crompton, C.J., et al., "'I Never Realised Everybody Felt as Happy as I Do When I Am Around Autistic People': A Thematic Analysis of Autistic Adults' Relationships with Autistic and Neurotypical Friends and Family," *Autism*, 26(6), 2020, 1438–48.

41. TheResearchAutism, *Simon Baron-Cohen Discusses ASD vs. ASC*, Video, December 14, 2014, www.youtube.com/watch?v=BDEHjLMOhHI

42. Baron-Cohen, *The Pattern Seekers*, 164.

43. Crawford, F., "Professor Temple Grandin Discusses the Most Personal Issue of Her Life: Autism," *Cornell Chronicle,* March 19, 2007, https://news.cornell.edu/stories

44. Samson, A, O. Huber, and W. Ruch, "Seven Decades After Hans Asperger's Observations: A Comprehensive Study of Humor in Individuals with Autism Spectrum Disorders," *Humor: International Journal of Humor Research*, 26, 2013, 441–60.

45. DDMH Lab, *Does This Make My Asperger's Look Big?* Michael McCreary, #TEDxYorkUSpectrum, Video, www.youtube.com/watch?v=jBVpgyIXllw

46. National Autistic Society, "Stories from the Spectrum: Bethany Black," n.d., autism.org.uk

47. Ewing, S., "I Have Asperger's: One of My Symptoms Included Being Obsessed with Ghosts': Under the Microscope with Dan Aykroyd," *Daily Mail,* December 9, 2013.

48. Gross, T., "Autism Spectrum Diagnosis Helped Comic Hannah Gadsby 'Be Kinder' to Herself," May 26, 2020, npr.org.

49. Oldenburg, A., 'Jerry Seinfeld: I'm on the Autism 'Spectrum,'" *USA Today*, November 7, 2014.

50. Samson, Huber, and Ruch, "Seven Decades After Hans Asperger's Observations," https://www.researchgate.net/publication/259366660_Seven_decades_after_Hans_Asperger's_observations_A_comprehensive_study_of_humor_in_individuals_with_Autism_Spectrum_Disorders

51. Rose, D., "*Do Autistic People 'Get' Jokes?*" *BBC News*, December 15, 2018.

52. Sansom, A., "Humour(lessness) Elucidated: Sense of Humor in Individuals with Autism Spectrum Disorders: Review and Introduction," *International Journal of Humor Research*, 26(3), 2013, 393–409.

53. Ledley, D.R., et al., "The Relationship Between Childhood Teasing and Later Interpersonal Functioning," *Journal of Psychopathology and Behavioral Assessment*, 28, 2006, 33–40.

54. Calleja, S., et al., "Healthcare Access for Autistic Adults: A Systematic Review," *Medicine*, 99(29), 2020, e20899.

55. Fusar-Poli, L., et al., "Missed Diagnoses and Misdiagnoses of Adults with Autism Spectrum Disorder, *European Archives of Psychiatry Clinical Neuroscience*, 272, 2020, 187–98.

56. Ibid.

57. Corden, K., R. Brewer, and E. Cage, "A Systematic Review of Healthcare Professionals' Knowledge, Self-Efficacy and Attitudes Towards Working with Autistic People," *Review Journal of Autism and Developmental Disorders,* 9, 2021, 386–99.

58. Fusar-Poli, et al., "Missed Diagnoses and Misdiagnoses," 187–98.

59. Calleja, et al., "Healthcare Access for Autistic Adults."

60. Stoddart, Burke, and King, *Asperger Syndrome in Adulthood*, 268.

61. Lawson, W., *Older Adults and Autism Spectrum Conditions: An Introduction and Guide*, Jessica Kingsley, 2015, 165.

62. Ibid.

63. National Joint Committee for the Communication Needs of Persons with Severe Disabilities, *Communication Bill of Rights*, n.d. Retrieved November 10, 2022, from www.asha.org/njc

64. Stoddart, Burke, and King, *Asperger Syndrome in Adulthood*, 102.

65. Donaldson, A.L., e. corbin, and J. McCoy, "'Everyone Deserves AAC': Preliminary Study of the Experiences of Speaking Autistic Adults Who Use Augmentative and Alternative Communication," *Perspectives of the ASHA Special Interest Groups, 6,* 2021, 315–26.

66. Ibid.

67. Volkmar, Reichow, and McPartland, *Adolescents and Adults with Autism Spectrum Disorder*, 232.

68. Tint, A., et al., "Correlates of Police Involvement among Adolescents and Adults with Autism Spectrum Disorder," *Journal of Autism and Developmental Disorders*, 47, 2017, 2639–47.

69. ASAN, *Colour Communication Badges.* Retrieved November 11, 2022 from https://autisticadvocacy.org

70. Muris, P., and T.H. Ollendick, "Selective Mutism and Its Relations to Social Anxiety Disorder and Autism Spectrum Disorder," *Clinical Child and Family Psychology Review*, 24, 2021, 294–325.

71. Attwood, *The Complete Guide to Asperger's Syndrome*, 70.

72. Carley, M.J., *Asperger's from the Inside Out: A Supportive and Practical Guide for Anyone with Asperger's Syndrome*, Penguin, 2008, 111.

73. Robison, J.E., *Look Me in the Eye*, Three Rivers Press, 2008, 243.

74. Attwood, *The Complete Guide to Asperger's Syndrome*, 127.

75. *Asperger's Syndrome: What Is Ongoing Traumatic Relationship Syndrome?* updated on March 17, 2022. Retrieved November 19, 2022, from https://psychcentral.com

76. ASAN, *ASAN's Response to Tony Attwood,* June 15, 2009. Retrieved November 19, 2022, from https://autisticadvocacy.org. I'm citing this for Tony Attwood's noting of Cassandra syndrome not being a diagnostic category. Having one of the world's top autism experts address this topic is relevant. While I personally share ASAN's dislike of FAAAS (Families of Adults Afflicted with Asperger's Syndrome), I do think their response to Attwood is over the top. This source is not linked for their opinion or as an endorsement of their opinion.

77. van Anders, S.M., "Testosterone and Sexual Desire in Healthy Women and Men," *Archives of Sexual Behavior*, 41(6), 2012, 1471–84.

78. Howard, P.L., and F. Sedgewick, "'Anything But the Phone!': Communication Mode Preferences in the Autism Community," *Autism*, 25(8), 2021, 2265–78.

79. Al-Nasrawi, R., "Online Dating, on the Autism Spectrum," *The Atlantic*, November 25, 2013.

80. Li, A.S., et al., "Exploring the Ability to Deceive in Children with Autism Spectrum Disorders," *Journal of Autism and Developmental Disorders*, 41(2), 2011, 185–95.

81. "Honouring the Culture of Autism," *Uniquely Human: The Podcast*, January 22, 2021. Retrieved November 11, 2022, from https://uniquelyhuman.com/2021/01/22/michael-john-carley

82. Lim, A., R.L. Young, and N. Brewer, "Autistic Adults May Be Erroneously Perceived as Deceptive and Lacking Credibility," *Journal of Autism and Developmental Disorders*, 52(2), 2022, 490–507.

83. Lewis, D., and H. Evans, "Is There a Link Between Whistleblowing and Autism?" Middlesex University London, May 4, 2021. Retrieved November 11, 2022, from https://mdxminds.com

84. Attwood, *The Complete Guide to Asperger's Syndrome*, 130.
85. Ibid., 129.
86. Ibid., 61.
87. Ibid., 130.
88. Frith, U., and Frith, C., "Reputation Management: In Autism, Generosity Is Its Own Reward," *Current Biology*, *21*(24), 2011, R994–5.
89. Howlin, *Autism and Asperger Syndrome*, 300.
90. Silberman, *NeuroTribes*, 17.
91. "Autreat Is Coming!" Autistic Self Advocacy Network, May 8, 2012.

## Chapter 4: Restricted and Repetitive Behaviours

1. Attwood, T., *The Complete Guide to Asperger's Syndrome*, 2nd ed., Jessica Kingsley Publishers, 2015, 185; Jolieffe, T., T. Landsdown, and T. Robinson, "Autism: A Personal Account," *Communication*, 26, 1992, 12–19.
2. Ambitious about Autism, *Meltdowns and Shutdowns,* n.d. Retrieved November 11, 2022, from www.ambitiousaboutautism.org.uk
3. Parents Action for Children, *How Can I Deal with an Autistic Meltdown*, n.d. Retrieved November 11, 2022, from https://parents.actionforchildren.org.uk
4. Rudy, L.J., "How Autistic Meltdowns Differ from Ordinary Temper Tantrums," *Verywell Health*, September 10, 2022. Retrieved November 20, 2022, from www.verywellhealth.com
5. Bottema-Beutel, K., et al., "Avoiding Ableist Language: Suggestions for Autism Researchers," *Autism in Adulthood*, 3(1), 2021, 18–29.
6. Laber-Warren, E., "The Benefits of Special Interests in Autism," *Spectrum,* May 12, 2021. Retrieved November 11, 2022, from www.spectrumnews.org
7. Kanner, "Autistic Disturbances," 217–250.
8. Attwood, *The Complete Guide to Asperger's Syndrome*, 184; Asperger, H., "'Autistic Psychopathy' in Childhood," in *Autism and Asperger Syndrome*, U. Frith, ed., Cambridge University Press, 1991, 72.
9. Attwood, *The Complete Guide to Asperger's Syndrome*, 184.
10. Silberman, *NeuroTribes,* 105.
11. Anthony, L.G., et al., "Interests in High-functioning Autism Are More Intense, Interfering, and Idiosyncratic Than Those in Neurotypical Development," *Development and Psychopathology*, 25(3), 2013, 643–52.
12. Attwood, *The Complete Guide to Asperger's Syndrome*, 185.
13. Stoddart, K., L. Burke, and R. King., *Asperger Syndrome in Adulthood: A Comprehensive Guide for Clinicians*, W.W. Norton, 2012, 64.
14. Attwood, *The Complete Guide to Asperger's Syndrome*, 192.
15. Stoddart, Burke, and King, *Asperger Syndrome in Adulthood*, 64.
16. Organization for Autism Research, "What Factors Impact the Work Performance of Adults with Autism," October 1, 2015; Kirchner, C.K., and I. Dziobek,

"Toward the Successful Employment of Adults with Autism: A First Analysis of Special Interests and Factors Deemed Important for Vocational Performance," *Scandinavian Journal of Child and Adolescent Psychiatry and Psychology*, 2(2), 2014, 77–85.

17. Ostrolenk, A., et al., "Hyperlexia: Systematic Review, Neurocognitive Modelling, and Outcome," *Neuroscience & Biobehavioral Reviews*, 79, 2017, 134–49.

18. McGill University, *Helping Children with Autism and Hyperlexia Learn to Understand What They Read: Q&A with Gigi Luk, Dianne Macdonald and Eve-Marie Quintin*, September 9, 2021. Retrieved November 12, 2022, from www.mcgill.ca/newsroom

19. Attwood, *The Complete Guide to Asperger's Syndrome*, 193.

20. Ibid.

21. Stoddart, Burke, and King, *Asperger Syndrome in Adulthood*, 64.

22. Bakker, T., et al., "Study Progression and Degree Completion of Autistic Students in Higher Education: A Longitudinal Study," *Higher Education*, 85, 2023, 1–26.

23. Attwood, *The Complete Guide to Asperger's Syndrome*, 251.

24. Stoddart, Burke, and King, *Asperger Syndrome in Adulthood*, 64, 211.

25. Tietz, J., "The Boy Who Loved Transit," *Harper's*, May 5, 2015.

26. Uljarević, M., et al., "Toward Better Characterization of Restricted and Unusual Interests in Youth with Autism," *Autism: The International Journal of Research and Practice*, 26(5), 2022, 1296–1304.

27. Kanner, "Autistic Disturbances," 219.

28. National Autistic Society, *Dealing with Change: A Guide for All Audiences*, n.d. Retrieved November 12, 2022, from www.autism.org.uk

29. The Onion, *Autistic Reporter, Michael Falk, Enchanted by Prison's Rigid Routine*, Video, November 21, 2011, www.youtube.com/watch?v=D04wb7P_v-4

30. Stoddart, Burke, and King, *Asperger Syndrome in Adulthood*, 64.

31. Attwood, *The Complete Guide to Asperger's Syndrome*, 93–94.

32. UNC School of Medicine, *Structured Teaching by TEACCH Staff*, n.d. Retrieved November 20, 2022, from https://teacch.com

33. Ibid.

34. Ibid.

35. Centers for Disease Control and Prevention, *Creating Structure and Rules*, n.d. Retrieved November 12, 2022, from www.cdc.gov

36. Fokkens-Burinsma, M., E.C.M. Van Rooij, and E.T. Canrinus, "Perceived Classroom Goal Structures as Predictors of Students' Personal Goals," *Teachers and Teaching, 26(1)*, 2020, 88–102.

37. Brenner, L.A., et al., "Time Reproduction Performance Is Associated with Age and Working Memory in High-Functioning Youth with Autism Spectrum Disorder," *Autism Research*, 8(1), 2015, 29–37.

38. Attwood, *The Complete Guide to Asperger's Syndrome*, 248.

39. Scott, M., et al., "Employers' Perception of the Costs and the Benefits of Hiring Individuals with Autism Spectrum Disorder in Open Employment in Australia," *PLOS ONE*, 12(5), 2017, e0177607.

40. Stoddart, Burke, and King, *Asperger Syndrome in Adulthood*, 89.

41. Not her real name.

42. Deweerdt, S., "Repetitive Behaviors and 'Stimming' in Autism, Explained," *Spectrum*, January 31, 2020. Retrieved November 12, 2022, from www.spectrumnews.org

43. U.S. House Government Reform Committee, *Vaccines and the Autism Epidemic: Reviewing the Federal Government's Track Record and Charting a Course for the Future*, December 10, 2002. Retrieved May 13, 2022, from www.congress.gov

44. Kapp, S.K., et al., "'People Should Be Allowed to Do What They Like': Autistic Adults' Views and Experiences of Stimming," *Autism*, *23*(7), 2019, 1782–92.

45. Moseley, R.L., et al., "Links Between Self-Injury and Suicidality in Autism," *Molecular Autism*, 11(1), 2020, 14; National Autistic Society, *Self-harm*, n.d. Retrieved November 12, 2022, from www.autism.org.uk

46. Zeliadt, N., "Sensory Sensitivity May Share Genetic Roots with Autism," *Spectrum*, January 17, 2018. Retrieved November 12, 2022, from www.spectrumnews.org

47. Marco, E.J., et al., "Sensory Processing in Autism: A Review of Neurophysiologic Findings," *Pediatric Research*, 69(5 Pt 2) 2011, 48R–54R.

48. Ibid.

49. Crane, L., L. Goddard, and L. Pring, "Sensory Processing in Adults with Autism Spectrum Disorders," *Autism*, 13(3), 2009, 215–28.

50. Williams, Z.J., et al., "Thermal Perceptual Thresholds Are Typical in Autism Spectrum Disorder but Strongly Related to Intra-individual Response Variability," *Scientific Reports*, 9, 2019, 12595.

51. Wenhart, T., et al., "Autistic Traits, Resting-State Connectivity, and Absolute Pitch in Professional Musicians: Shared and Distinct Neural Features," *Molecular Autism*, 10, 2019, 20.

52. Hughes, V., "Autism Often Accompanied by 'Super Vision,' Studies Find," *Spectrum*, December 9, 2009. Retrieved November 12, 2022, from www.spectrumnews.org

53. Herrmann, M., "How Public Attractions Are Better Accommodating Guests with Sensory Needs," *Forbes*, October 26, 2018.

54. Breen, K., "Magazine Names Channel-Port aux Basques Most Autism-Friendly Town in Canada," *CBCNews*, April 3, 2018. Retrieved November 12, 2022, from www.cbc.ca/news

55. Autism Society of America, Resources: Employment, n.d., Retrieved November 12, 2022, from https://autismsociety.org/resources/employment/

56. Happé, F. and U. Frith, "The Weak Coherence Account: Detail-Focused Cognitive Style in Autism Spectrum Disorders," *Journal of Autism and Developmental Disorders*, 36(1), 2006, 5–25.

57. Baron-Cohen, S., et al., "Talent in Autism: Hyper-Systemizing, Hyper-Attention to Detail and Sensory Hypersensitivity," *Philosophical Transactions: Biological Sciences*, 364(1522), 2009, 1377–83.

58. Koldewyn, K., et al., "Global/Local Processing in Autism: Not a Disability, but a Disinclination," *Journal of Autism and Developmental Disorders* 43(10), 2013, 2329–40.

59. Demetriou, E.A., M.M. DeMayo, and A.J. Guastella, "Executive Function in Autism Spectrum Disorder: History, Theoretical Models, Empirical Findings, and Potential as an Endophenotype," *Frontiers in Psychiatry*, 10, 2019, 753.

60. Stoddart, Burke, and King, *Asperger Syndrome in Adulthood*, 160.

61. Demetriou, DeMayo, and Guastella, "Executive Function in Autism Spectrum Disorder."

62. Howlin, P., *Autism and Asperger Syndrome: Preparing for Adulthood*, 2nd ed., Routledge Taylor and Francis Group, 2004, 73.

63. Ibid.

64. Ibid.

65. *Autism, PDD-NOS & Asperger's fact sheets, Echolalia, Autism and Intervention Strategies for Parents*, n.d. Retrieved April 30, 2023, from www.autism-help.org

66. Cravedi, E., et al., "Tourette Syndrome and Other Neurodevelopmental Disorders: A Comprehensive Review," *Child and Adolescent Psychiatry and Mental Health*, 11, 2017, 59.

67. Volkmar, Reichow, and McPartland, *Adolescents and Adults with Autism Spectrum Disorder*, 23.

68. Nemours KidsHealth, *Speech-Language Therapy*, n.d. Retrieved November 12, 2022, from https://kidshealth.org

69. Ebbels, S.H, et al., "Effectiveness of 1:1 Speech and Language Therapy for Older Children with (Developmental) Language Disorder," *International Journal of Language and Communication Disorders*, 52(4), 2017, 528–39.

## Chapter 5: An Issue of Data

1. Geneva Centre for Autism, *Autism in Adulthood: What We Do and Don't Know*, Video, March 22, 2016, www.youtube.com/watch?v=bilTru-Ah4s

2. Fombonne, E., "Camouflage and Autism," *Journal of Child Psychology and Psychiatry*, 61(7), 2020, 735–38.

3. Lai, M.C., et al., "'Camouflaging' in Autistic People: Reflection on Fombonne (2020)," *Journal of Child Psychology and Psychiatry*, *62*(8), 2021.

4. Tantam, D., "Aging and Autism Spectrum Disorder: Experiential and Social Perspectives," in *Autism Spectrum Disorder in Mid and Later Life*, S.D. Wright, ed., Jessica Kingsley, 2015, 107.

5. Ibid., 108.

6. Di Cicco, M.E., V. Ragazzo, and T. Jacinto, "Mortality in Relation to Smoking," *Breathe* (Sheff), 12(3), 2016, 275–6.

7. Volkmar, Reichow, and McPartland, *Adolescents and Adults with Autism Spectrum Disorder*, 76.

8. Brugha, T., et al., "Epidemiology of Autism Spectrum Disorders in Adults in the Community in England," *Archives of General Psychiatry*, 68(5), 2011, 459–65.

9. Brugha, T.S., et al., "Epidemiology of Autism in Adults Across Age Groups and Ability Levels, *British Journal of Psychiatry*, 209(6), 2016, 498–503.

10. Brugha et al., "Epidemiology of Autism Spectrum Disorders," 439.

11. Ibid.

12. Arnold, S., et al., "Cohort Profile: The Australian Longitudinal Study of Adults with Autism," *BMJ Open*, 9, 2019, e030798.

13. *Research*, n.d. Retrieved November 12, 2022, from https://teacch.com/research

14. Tantam, "Aging and Autism Spectrum Disorder," 108.

15. Stenson, J., "Why the Focus of Autism Research Is Shifting Away from Searching for a 'Cure,'" *ABCNews*, September 29, 2019.

16. *Research*, n.d. Retrieved November 12, 2022, from https://autisticadvocacy.org

17. *Autism Genome Project*, n.d. Retrieved November 12, 2022, from https://genomecanada.ca

18. As an example, K. Bottema-Beutel et al., "Avoiding Ableist Language: Suggestions for Autism Researchers," *Autism in Adulthood*, 3(1), 2021.

19. Autism Canada, *Summary Report: Aging and Autism, A Think Tank Round Table, 2018.* Retrieved August 9, 2023, from https://autismalberta.ca/wp-content/uploads/2023/03/Aging_-Autism_-A_Think_Tank_Round_Table.pdf

20. Arkowitz, H., and S.O. Lilienfield, "Is There Really an Autism Epidemic?" *Scientific American*, August 1, 2012. I should note that I do not agree with the definition of autism presented in this source. It is much too narrow and much too focused on "severe" cases. It merely shows that autism has been called an epidemic.

21. "Hot Topics in Autism Research, 2020," *Spectrum*, December 23, 2020. Retrieved November 12, 2022, from www.spectrumnews.org

22. Mason, D., et al., "Older Age Autism Research: A Rapidly Growing Field, but Still a Long Way to Go," *Autism in Adulthood*, *4*(2), 2022, 164–72.

23. Volkmar, Reichow, and McPartland, *Adolescents and Adults with Autism Spectrum Disorder*, 2; Geneva Centre for Autism, *Autism in Adulthood* (1:01:37)

24. *Autism Spectrum Disorder in Mid and Later Life*, Jessica Kingsley, 2015, 15.

25. Autism Canada, *Summary Report*, 3, 20.

26. Ibid.

27. Ratcliffe, A., *Our Autistic Lives: Personal Accounts from Autistic Adults from Around the World Ages 20 to 70+*, Jessica Kingsley, 2020.

28. Wake W., E. Endlich, and R. Lagos, *Older Autistic Adults in Their Own Words: The Lost Generation*, AAPC, 2021.

## Chapter 6: An Issue of Resources and Employment

1. Rogge, N., and J. Janssen, "The Economic Costs of Autism Spectrum Disorder: A Literature Review," *Journal of Autism and Developmental Disorders*, 49(7), 2019, 2873–900.

2. Holland Bloorview Kids Rehabilitation Hospital, *The Dad Behind Carly's Voice*, Video, November 11, 2013, www.youtube.com/watch?v=MKFP_1J6QjU

3. Lowinger, S., and S. Pearlman-Avnion, *Autism in Adulthood*, Springer, 2019, 134–35.

4. Autism Research Centre, *The Eindhoven Study: STEM Regions and Autism*, n.d. Retrieved November 12, 2022, from www.autismresearchcentre.com

5. Wei, X., et al., "Science, Technology, Engineering, and Mathematics (STEM) Participation Among College Students with an Autism Spectrum Disorder," *Journal of Autism and Developmental Disorders*, 43(7), 2013, 1539–46.

6. Bureau of Labour Statistics, *May 2021 National Occupational Employment and Wage Estimates*. Retrieved November 12, 2022, from www.bls.gov

7. More detail on this can be found in chapter 8, An Issue of Self-Understanding.

8. Much of the information in this section came directly from the Ontario Ministry of Children, Community, and Social Services. Thank you for your help.

9. *Closing Institutions for People with a Developmental Disability*, March 31, 2009. Retrieved November 12, 2022, from https://news.ontario.ca

10. Ibid.

11. Corbett, R., "After the Institutions: Why Ontario's Decision to Shut Long-Term Care Facilities Haunts Some to This Day," *Ottawa Citizen*, November 25, 2016.

12. Financial Accountability Office of Ontario, *Autism Services: A Financial Review of Autism Services and Program Design Considerations for the New Ontario Autism Program*, July 21, 2020, fao-on.ca

13. Parliament of Canada, *Bill C-360: An Act to Amend the Canada Health Act (Autism Spectrum Disorder)*, n.d., https://www.parl.ca/LegisInfo/en/bill/40-3/c-360

14. Canadian Press, "Ontario Budget 2022: Highlights from the Ford Government's Pre-Election Pitch," *CBC News*, April 28, 2022.

15. McQuigge, M., "What Exactly Is Ontario's New Autism Program? A Look at the Controversy It Has Created," *GlobalNews,* February 25, 2019. Retrieved November 12, 2022, from https://globalnews.ca/news

16. Jones, A., "Ontario Overhauls Autism Program to Clear Waiting List of 23,000 Children," *National Post,* February 6, 2019.

17. Crawley, M., "Ford Government Pledges to Clear Autism Therapy Waitlist, Provide Cash to Families in Need," *CBC News,* February 6, 2020. Retrieved November 12, 2022, from www.cbc.ca/news

18. McQuigge, "What Exactly Is Ontario's New Autism Program?"

19. *Ontario Autism Program: Childhood Budgets*, n.d. Retrieved November 12, 2022, from www.ontario.ca

20. McQuigge, "What Exactly Is Ontario's New Autism Program?"

21. Statistics Canada, *Canadian Income Survey, 2020*, March 23, 2022. Retrieved November 12, 2022, from www150.statcan.gc.ca; Government of Ontario, *Ontario Increasing Access to Services for Children with Autism*, December 3, 2021. Retrieved November 12, 2022, from https://news.ontario.ca/en/release/1001279/ontario-increasing-access-to-services-for-children-with-autism

22. Jones, A., "Slow Progress in Ontario Autism Program Rollout: Officials Insist They're on Target," *Toronto CityNews,*, August 13, 2022. Retrieved November 12, 2022, from https://toronto.citynews.ca

23. Canadian Press, "Ontario Autism Services Waitlist Grew to 27,600 Children in 2019–2020," *ctv News*, July 21, 2020. Retrieved November 12, 2022, from https://toronto.ctvnews.ca

24. Government of Ontario, *Ontario Increasing Access to Services.*

25. Sharp, M., "Ontario Budget Watchdog Says Ford Government's Autism Plan Falls Short," *National Observer*, July 21, 2020.

26. The Agenda with Steve Paikin, *Managing Ontario's Autism Services*, Video, February 26, 2019, www.youtube.com/watch?v=EMZAEkKmEzM&t=673s

27. Elsiufi, R., "What Ontario's Major Parties Are Offering for Autism Funding," *cbc News*, May 17, 2022. Retrieved November 13, 2022, from www.cbc.ca/news

28. The Agenda with Steve Paikin. *Managing Ontario's Autism Services.*

29. Jones, A., "Ontario ndp Promises Universal Mental Health Care at a Cost of $1.15B a Year," *cbcNews*, April 3, 2022. Retrieved November 13, 2022, from www.cbc.ca/news

30. Ontario Medical Association, *Medical Organizations Call for New Funding and Editions*, April 3, 2022. Retrieved November 13, 2022, from www.oma.org

31. Freeman, T.R., et al., "Shifting Tides in the Emigration Patterns of Canadian Physicians to the United States: A Cross-Sectional Secondary Data Analysis," *bmc Health Services Research*, 16(1), 2016, 678.

32. Statista, *Number of Canadians That Are Enrolled in Private Prescription Drug Plans in 2020, by Province*, n.d. Retrieved November 13, 2022, from www.statista.com

33. Florida Atlantic University, *Fact Sheet-Discrete Trial*, n.d. Retrieved November 13, 2022, from www.fau.edu/education

34. aba Made Easy, *aba Therapy: The First Sessions of Therapy*, Video, June 22, 2015, www.youtube.com/watch?v=SWmEe5QPDo8

35. Cherry, K., "What is aba Therapy?," *Verywell Mind*, July 4, 2021. Retrieved November 13, 2022, from www.verywellmind.com

36. Makrygianni, M.K., et al., "The Effectiveness of Applied Behavior Analytic Interventions for Children with Autism Spectrum Disorder: A Meta-Analytic Study," *Research in Autism Spectrum Disorders*, 51, 2018, 18–31; Leaf, J.B., et al., "Concerns About aba-Based Intervention: An Evaluation and Recommendations," *Journal of Autism and Developmental Disorders*, 52, 2022, 2838–53.

37. Kennedy Krieger Institute, *Scientific Support for Applied Behavior Analysis from the Neurobehavioral Unit (nbu)*, n.d. Retrieved November 13, 2022, from www.kennedykrieger.org

38. Lovaas, O.I., and T. Smith, "Intensive Behavioral Treatment for Young Autistic Children," in *Advances in Clinical Child Psychology*, 11, B.B. Lahey and A.E. Kazdin, eds., Springer, 1988.

39. Shkedy, G., D. Shkedy, and A.H. Sandoval-Norton, "Long-term aba Therapy Is Abusive: A Response to Gorycki, Ruppel, and Zane," *Advances in Neurodevelopmental Disorders*, 5, 2021, 126–34.

40. Kirkham, P., "'The Line Between Intervention and Abuse': Autism and Applied Behaviour Analysis," *History of the Human Sciences*, 30(2), 2017, 107–26.

41. ASAN, *#StopTheShock: The Judge Rotenberg Center, Torture, and How We Can Stop It*, n.d. Retrieved November 13, 2022, from https://autisticadvocacy.org/actioncenter/issues/school/climate/jrc/

42. The Agenda with Steve Paikin, *Managing Ontario's Autism Services.*

43. ABA Learning Centre, *What Is the Number of Recommended Hours of Intervention per Week?* n.d. Retrieved November 13, 2022, from https://abacentre.ca/faqs

44. Business Wire, *The U.S. Autism Treatment Market Is Expected to Reach $2.23 Billion by 2022*, May 1, 2018. Retrieved November 13, 2022, from www.businesswire.com/news

45. Binns, A.V., et al., "Looking Back and Moving Forward: A Scoping Review of Research on Preschool Autism Interventions in the Field of Speech-Language Pathology," *Autism & Developmental Language Impairments*, 6, 2021.

46. Group Enroll, *The Cost of Speech Therapy Sessions in Canada*, July 29, 2022. Retrieved November 13, 2022, from https://groupenroll.ca/the-cost-of-speech-therapy-sessions-in-canada/

47. Geretsegger, M., et al., "Music Therapy for People with Autism Spectrum Disorder," *Cochrane Database of Systematic Reviews*, 6, 2014, CD004381.

48. Howlin, P., *Autism and Asperger Syndrome: Preparing for Adulthood*, 2nd ed., Routledge Taylor and Francis Group, 2004, 54–55. Facilitated communication is a technique where a person, called a facilitator, guides an autistic person's hand to help them write their thoughts through writing or typing. This technique has been discredited in the scientific community.

49. Travers, J., "Psuedoscience, Science, and Decision Making in Autism Education Programs," Lecture, Penn State National Autism Conference, August 5, 2021.

50. Nicolaidis, C., C.C. Kripke, and D. Raymaker, "Primary Care for Adults on the Autism Spectrum, *Medical Clinics of North America*, 98(5), 2014, 1169–91. This source does not explicitly say that autistic adults are more often given developmental rather than ABA-based treatment, but their summary of interventions lists several non-ABA programs.

51. *How Can Applied Behavior Analysts Help Adults with Autism?* n.d. Retrieved November 20, 2022, from www.appliedbehavioranalysisprograms.com/faq

52. Vick, B., K. Jones, and S. Mitra, "Poverty and Psychiatric Diagnosis in the U.S.: Evidence from the Medical Expenditure Panel Survey," *Journal of Mental Health Policy and Economics, 15*(2), 2012.

53. *Is Therapy Covered by OHIP?* n.d. Retrieved November 20, 2022, from https://everwellcounselling.ca

54. *Psychotherapy Fees*, n.d. Retrieved November 14, 2022, from https://therapytoronto.ca

55. Frith, U., *Autism: Explaining the Enigma*, 2nd ed., Blackwell, 2003, 13.

56. *Lorna Wing Centre for Autism*, n.d. Retrieved November 13, 2022, from www.autismconnect.com/directory

57. Robison, J.E., *Look Me in the Eye*, Crown, 2008, 237.

58. This fact was given to me by the Ministry of Children, Community, and Social Services.

59. Government of Ontario, *Income Support from ODSP*, n.d. Retrieved November 19, 2022, from www.ontario.ca; Government of Ontario, *Definition and Treatment of Assets*, n.d. Retrieved November 19, 2022, from www.ontario.ca

60. Government of Ontario, *Ontario Disability Support Program*, n.d. Retrieved November 19, 2022, from www.ontario.ca

61. Ibid.

62. Government of Canada, *Disability Tax Credit (DTC)*, n.d. Retrieved November 13, 2022, from www.canada.ca/en/revenue-agency

63. Government of Canada, *Registered Disability Savings Plan (RDSP)*, n.d. Retrieved November 19, 2022, from www.canada.ca/en/revenue-agency

64. RBC, *Henson Trusts*, n.d. Retrieved November 19, 2022, from https://ca.rbcwealthmanagement.com

65. DSO, *Passport Program: Funding for Community Participation Services and Supports*. Retrieved November 19, 2022, from www.dsontario.ca/passport-program

66. Government of Canada, *National Action Plan to End Gender-Based Violence Backgrounder*, n.d. Retrieved November 13, 2022, from https://www.canada.ca/en/women-gender-equality/news/2022/11/national-action-plan-to-end-gender-based-violence-backgrounder.html

67. Autism Ontario, *Introducing the Top Five Priorities for Autism in Ontario*, October 5, 2020. Retrieved November 13, 2022, from www.autismontario.com/news

68. Autism Ontario, *Improving Social Skills Interventions for Ontarians with Autism Spectrum Disorder*, October 5, 2020. Retrieved November 13, 2022, from www.autismontario.com

69. DSO, *Housing*, n.d. Retrieved November 19, 2022, from https://www.dsontario.ca/housing

70. Government of Ontario, *Developmental Services Waitlist Report*, n.d. Retrieved November 19, 2022, from https://data.ontario.ca

71. Slaughter, G., "Group Homes for Adults with Autism Unaffordable and Inaccessible, Parents Say," *CTV News*, June 8, 2016. Retrieved November 19, 2022, from www.ctvnews.ca

72. Donovan K., "Adults Beaten in Group Homes: Hundreds of Cases May Just Be Tip of Iceberg," *Toronto Star*, October 28, 2001.

73. Russell, A., et al., "Inspection Reports Reveal Disturbing Conditions Inside Ontario Group Homes," *Global News*, June 1, 2022. Retrieved November 19, 2022, from https://globalnews.ca/news

74. Dudley, C., and J.H. Emery, *The Value of Caregiver Time: Costs of Support and Care for Individuals Living with Autism Spectrum Disorder*, University of Calgary School of Public Policy SPP Research Papers, 7*(1), 2014.*

75. Walters, S., M. Loades, and A.J. Russell, "A Systematic Review of Effective Modifications to Cognitive Behavioural Therapy for Young People with Autism

Spectrum Disorders," *Review Journal of Autism and Developmental Disorders*, 3, 2016, 137–53.

76. Public Health Agency of Canada, *A Dementia Strategy for Canada: Together We Aspire*, 2019. Retrieved November 19, 2022, from https://alzheimer.ca/sites/default/files/documents

77. Government of Canada, *National Action Plan to End Gender-Based Violence Backgrounder*.

78. UK Government, *National Strategy for Autistic Children, Young People and Adults: 2021 to 2026*, July 21, 2021. Retrieved November 19, 2022, from www.gov.uk/government/publications

79. Scottish Government, *Scottish Strategy for Autism: Evaluation*, September 24, 2021. Retrieved November 21, 2022, from www.gov.scot/publications; Department of Health, *Autism Strategy and Action Plan*, n.d. Retrieved November 21, 2022, from www.health-ni.gov.uk; Autism Europe, *Spanish Strategy for Autism Spectrum Disorder*, Presentation, n.d. Retrieved November 21, 2022, from www.autismeurope.org; *Malta National Autism Strategy 2021–2030*, March 30, 2021. Retrieved November 21, 2022, from https://meae.gov

80. Canadian Academy of Health Sciences, *Autism in Canada: Considerations for Future Public Policy Development*, n.d. Retrieved November 19, 2022, from https://cahs-acss.ca

81. Autism Alliance of Canada, *Working Together to Advance a National Autism Strategy*, n.d. Retrieved November 19, 2022, from www.autismalliance.ca

82. A4A Ontario, *Canadian Autistic Self-Advocacy Groups Oppose CASDA's National Autism Strategy*, October 8, 2019. Retrieved November 20, 2022, from https://a4aontario.com

83. CASDA, *Blueprint for a National Autism Spectrum Disorder Strategy: How the Federal Government Can Lead*, March 1, 2019. Retrieved November 20, 2022, from www.autismalliance.ca

84. *Policy Compendium*, March 1, 2019. Retrieved November 20, 2022, from www.autismalliance.ca

85. Health Canada, *Canada Health Act Annual Report 2014–2015*, n.d. Retrieved November 20, 2022, from www.canada.ca

86. Public Health Agency of Canada, *A Dementia Strategy for Canada*.

87. Standing Senate Committee on Social Affairs, Science and Technology, *Final Report on: The Enquiry on the Funding for the Treatment of Autism, Pay Now or Pay Later Autism Families in Crisis*, March 1, 2007. Retrieved November 21, 2022, from https://publications.gc.ca

88. A4A Ontario, *Canadian Autistic Self-Advocacy Groups Oppose CASDA's National Autism Strategy*.

89. Parliament of Canada, *Bill S-203: An Act Respecting a Federal Framework on Autism Spectrum Disorder*, October 17, 2022. Retrieved November 21, 2022, from https://www.parl.ca/legisinfo/en/bill/44-1/s-203

90. Ibid. Retrieved May 3, 2023, from https://www.parl.ca/legisinfo/en/bill/44-1/s-203

91. National Council on Aging (ACO), *SSI vs. SSDI: The Differences, Benefits, and How to Apply*, March 16, 2022. Retrieved November 21, 2022, from https://ncoa.org

92. Social Security Administration, *If I Get Married, Will It Affect My Benefits?* n.d. Retrieved November 21, 2022, from https://faq.ssa.gov

93. Rock, J., "Twenty Years of Marriage Equality? No, Not for Disabled Ontarians," *Toronto Star*, January 13, 2021; Government of Ontario, "*2.3-Spouse*," n.d. Retrieved November 21, 2022, from www.ontario.ca

94. Garbero, G., "Rights Not Fundamental: Disability and the Right to Marry," *Saint Louis University Journal of Health Law & Policy*, *14*(2), 2021.

95. AHRC New York City, "Marriage Proposal Carries Consequences," *Autism Spectrum News*, September 29, 2022, https://autismspectrumnews.org/marriage-proposal-carries-consequences/; Rock, "Twenty Years of Marriage Equality?"

96. *Marriage Access for People with Special Abilities Act*, H.R.1529, 116th Cong. (2019). Retrieved November 21, 2022, from https://www.congress.gov/bill/116th-congress/house-bill/1529

97. Gurbuz, E., M. Hanley, and D.M. Riby, "University Students with Autism: The Social and Academic Experiences of University in the UK," *Journal of Autism and Developmental Disorders*, 49, 2019, 617–31.

98. Ontario Human Rights Commission, *Accommodating Students with Disabilities: Roles and Responsibilities (Fact Sheet)*, www.ohrc.on.ca

99. Manett, J., "Somewhere in the Middle: Understandings of Friendship and Approaches to Social Engagement Among Postsecondary Students with Autism Spectrum Disorder," Doctoral dissertation, University of Toronto, 2020, 2.

100. Ibid.

101. Statista, *Number of Students Enrolled in Postsecondary Institutions in Canada in 2019/20, by Province*, November 1, 2021. Retrieved November 21, 2022, from https://www.statista.com/statistics/447802/enrollment-of-postsecondary-students-in-canada-by-province/

102. Manett, "Somewhere in the Middle," 112.

103. National Autistic Society, *New Shocking Data Highlights the Autism Employment Gap*, February 21, 2021. Retrieved November 21, 2022, from www.autism.org.uk; Simmons, T. "86% of Adults with Autism Are Unemployed: This Job Fair Aims to Change That," *CBC News*, April 9, 2019, www.cbc.ca/news/canada

104. Volkmar, Reichow, and McPartland, *Adolescents and Adults with Autism Spectrum Disorders*, 48.

105. Ontario Human Rights Commission, *Policy and Guidelines on Disability and the Duty to Accommodate*, revised November 23, 2000. Retrieved November 21, 2022, from www.ohrc.on.ca

106. Government of Ontario, *The Path to 2025: Ontario's Accessibility Action Plan*, n.d. Retrieved November 21, 2022, from www.ontario.ca

107. Swartz, M., "Benefits of Hiring People on the Autism Spectrum," n.d. Retrieved November 21, 2022, from https://hiring.monster.ca/resources; Enna, *7 Benefits of Employing Autistic Individuals*, n.d. Retrieved November 21, 2022, from https://enna.org/7-benefits-of-employing-autistic-individuals/

108. Geneva Centre for Autism, *Evening and Weekend Respite,* n.d. Retrieved November 21, 2022, from www.autism.net; Autistics United Canada, *Events*, n.d. Retrieved November 21, 2022, from www.autisticsunitedca.org

109. Drexel University, *Systemic Challenges to Implementing Universal Basic Income*, 2022. Retrieved November 21, 2022, from https://drexel.edu

## Chapter 7: An Issue of Public Understanding

1. Moya, M.J., "Autism Acceptance Month Is Underway: Here's Why the Name Is Important," *USA Today*, April 2, 2022.

2. Alsehemi, M.A., et al., "Public Awareness of Autism Spectrum Disorder," *Neurosciences* (Riyadh, Saudi Arabia), 22(3), 2017, 213–15.

3. Kuzminski, R., et al., "Linking Knowledge and Attitudes: Determining Neurotypical Knowledge About and Attitudes Towards Autism," *PLOS ONE*, 14(7), 2019, e0220197.

4. Dickie, G., "Why Polls Were Mostly Wrong," *Scientific American*, November 13, 2020.

5. Yu, L., S. Stronach, and A.J. Harrison, "Public Knowledge and Stigma of Autism Spectrum Disorder: Comparing China with the United States," *Autism: The International Journal of Research and Practice*, 24(6), 2020, 1531–45.

6. Chen, W.J., et al., "Autism Spectrum Disorders: Prenatal Genetic Testing and Abortion Decision-Making Among Taiwanese Mothers of Affected Children," *International Journal of Environmental Research and Public Health*, 17(2), 2020, 476.

7. Alsehemi, et al., "Public Awareness of Autism Spectrum Disorder," 213-15.

8. Effatpanah, M., et al., "A Preliminary Survey of Autism Knowledge and Attitude Among Health Care Workers and Pediatricians in Tehran, Iran," *Iranian Journal of Child Neurology*, 13(2), 2019, 29–35.

9. PooranLaw, *Ontario Considers Expanding Definition of 'Child' in Children's Law Reform Act to Include Adult 'Children' with Disabilities*, January 8, 2021. Retrieved August 9, 2023, from https://pooranlaw.com/ontario-considers-expanding-definition-of-child-in-childrens-law-reform-act-to-include-adult-children-with-disabilities/; A4A Ontario, *Ontario May Change Legal Definition of 'Child' in Legislation to Include Disabled Adults: A4A Responds*, January 2, 2021. Retrieved November 21, 2022, from https://a4aontario.com

10. Government of Ontario, *Substitute Decisions Act, 1992, S.O. 1992, c. 30.* Retrieved November 21, 2022, from www.ontario.ca/laws/statute/92s30

11. United Nations Human Rights: Office of the High Commissioner, *Discrimination Against Autistic Persons: The Rule Rather Than the Exception, UN Rights Experts*, April 1, 2015. Retrieved November 21, 2022, from www.ohchr.org/en/press-releases

12. Sasson, N.J., et al., "Neurotypical Peers Are Less Willing to Interact with Those with Autism Based on Thin Slice Judgments, *Scientific Reports*, 7, 2017, 40700.

13. Mattson, M.P. "Superior Pattern Processing Is the Essence of the Evolved Human Brain," *Frontiers in Neuroscience*, 8, 2014, 265.

14. Gemegah, E., D. Hartas, and V. Totsika, "Public Attitudes to People with ASD: Contact, Knowledge and Ethnicity," *Advances in Autism*, 7(3), 2021, 225–40.

15. Vincent, J., "Employability for UK University Students and Graduates on the Autism Spectrum: Mobilities and Materialities," *Scandinavian Journal of Disability Research*, 22(1), 2020, 12–24.

16. Vincent cites numerous studies in the part of this quote after the ellipses: M. Adolfsson and A. Simmeborn Fleischer, "Applying the ICF to Identify Requirements for Students with Asperger Syndrome in Higher Education," *Developmental Neurorehabilitation*, 18(3), 2015, 190–202; S.L. Jackson, J.L. Hart, and F.R. Volkmar, "Preface: Special Issue, College Experiences for Students with Autism Spectrum Disorder," *Journal of Autism and Developmental Disorders*, 48(3), 2018, 639–42; Association of Graduate Careers Advisory Services, "What Happens Next? 2018 Report, 2019," accessed November 3, 2022, www.agcas.org.uk

17. Romualdez A.M., B. Heasman, Z. Walker, J. Davies, and A. Remington, "'People Might Understand Me Better': Diagnostic Disclosure Experience of Autistic Individuals in the Workplace," *Autism in Adulthood*, 3(2), 2021, 157–67.

18. Government of Canada, "Equality Rights - Section 15," in *Guide to the Charter of Rights and Freedoms*, n.d. Retrieved November 12, 2022, from https://www.canada.ca; As an example of other countries, the U.S. prohibits disability on discrimination based on the ADA: Department of Labor, *Employment Laws: Disability & Discrimination*, n.d. Retrieved November 12, 2022, from www.dol.gov

19. Praslova, L.N., "Autism Doesn't Hold People Back at Work. Discrimination Does," *Harvard Business Review,* December 13, 2021. Retrieved November 12, 2022, from www.dol.gov

20. Heasman, B., "Employers May Discriminate Against Autism Without Realising," *London School of Economics* (blog), August 10, 2017. Retrieved November 12, 2022, from https://blogs.lse.ac.uk

21. Ibid.

22. AUsome Training, *Autism Training for Professionals*, n.d. Retrieved November 21, 2022, from https://ausometraining.com

23. Kerry's Place, *Autism Spectrum Disorder Job Readiness Program*, n.d. Retrieved November 21, 2022, from www.kerrysplace.org, Full disclosure, I used to volunteer at Kerry's Place in their musical program, swimming program, and hang-out program.

24. Autism Ontario, *Fair Jobs. Equal Employment. Inclusive Workplaces,* n.d., Retrieved November 21, 2022, from www.autismontario.com

25. Canucks Autism Network, *Employment Programs & Services*, n.d. Retrieved November 21, 2022, from www.canucksautism.ca

26. Autism Society, *Employment*, n.d. Retrieved November 21, 2022, from www.autism-society.org

27. National Autism Society, *Autistic Fatigue: A Guide for Autistic Adults*. Retrieved November 21, 2022, from www.autism.org.uk

28. Waisman, T., et al., Free for Life International Presents: The Conference on Autism and Human Trafficking, Panel discussion, April 28, 2021, https://www.watraffickinghelp.org/new-events/2021/4/28/conference-on-autism-and-human-trafficking

29. Morin, A., *What Is Universal Design for Learning (UDL)?* n.d. Retrieved November 21, 2022, from www.understood.org

30. Generation Next, *Could It Be Asperger's?*, video, January 25, 2015, www.youtube.com/watch?v=LuZFThlOiJI

31. Rowland, S., "School Improvement for Autistic Pupils," National Autistic Society, May 11, 2021. Retrieved November 21, 2022, from www.autism.org.uk

32. "Autistic Advocacy: An Interview with Julia Bascom," March 26, 2021. Retrieved November 21, 2022, from https://uniquelyhuman.com/2021/03/26/autistic-advocacy-julia-bascom/

33. Sanz-Cervera, P., et al., "The Effectiveness of TEACCH Intervention in Autism Spectrum Disorder: A Review Study," *Papeles del Psicólogo, 39*(1), 2018, 40–50.

34. Attwood, T., *The Complete Guide to Asperger's Syndrome*, 2nd ed., Jessica Kingsley Publishers, 2015, 325.

35. Cage, E., J. Di Monaco, and V. Newell, "Experiences of Autism Acceptance and Mental Health in Autistic Adults," *Journal of Autism and Developmental Disorders*, 48(2), 2018, 473–84.

36. Volkmar, Reichow, and McPartland, *Adolescents and Adults with Autism Spectrum Disorders*, 29.

37. Ibid.

38. Organization for Autism Research, *Sibling Support*, n.d. Retrieved November 21, 2022, from https://researchautism.org/families/sibling-support/

39. Kerry's Place, *All About You: A Support Group for Siblings*, n.d. Retrieved November 21, 2022, from www.kerrysplace.org

40. *Sibling Support Project*, n.d. Retrieved November 21, 2022, from https://siblingsupport.org

41. Senate of Canada, *Human Rights Committee to Study the Forced and Coerced Sterilization of Persons in Canada*, March 27, 2119. Retrieved May 5, 2023, from https://sencanada.ca/en/newsroom; Roy, A., A. Roy, and M. Roy, "The Human Rights of Women with Intellectual Disability," *Journal of the Royal Society of Medicine*, 105(9), 2012, 384–89.

42. National Women's Law Center, *Forced Sterilization of Disabled People in the United States*, February 7, 2022. Retrieved May 5, 2023, from https://nwlc.org/resource

43. Mair, M.L., "The Right to Procreate: Intellectual Disability and the Law," *Australian College of Midwives Inc. Journal*, 5(4), 1992, 16–20.

44. Pohl, A.L., et al., "A Comparative Study of Autistic and Non-Autistic Women's Experience of Motherhood," *Molecular Autism*, 11(1), 2020, 3.

45. Attwood, *The Complete Guide to Asperger's Syndrome*, 325.

46. Volkmar, Reichow, and McPartland, *Adolescents and Adults with Autism Spectrum Disorders*, 64.

## Chapter 8: An Issue of Self-Understanding

1. Williams, D. *Nobody Nowhere: The Extraordinary Autobiography of an Autistic*, Avon Books, 40.

2. Sacks O., *An Anthropologist from Mars*, Vintage Canada, 1996, 259.

3. Lai, M.C., and S. Baron-Cohen, "Identifying the Lost Generation of Adults with Autism Spectrum Conditions," *Lancet*, 2(11), 2015, 1013–27.

4. "Honouring the Culture of Autism," *Uniquely Human: The Podcast,* January 22, 2021. Retrieved November 11, 2022, from https://uniquelyhuman.com/2021/01/22/michael-john-carley

5. Ragelienė, T., "Links of Adolescents Identity Development and Relationship with Peers: A Systematic Literature Review," *Journal of the Canadian Academy of Child and Adolescent Psychiatry*, 25(2), 2016, 97–105.

6. Howlin, P., *Autism and Asperger Syndrome: Preparing for Adulthood*, 2nd ed., Routledge Taylor and Francis Group, 2004, 37; ibid., chapter 4.

7. Carley, M.J., *Asperger's from the Inside Out: A Supportive and Practical Guide for Anyone with Asperger's Syndrome*, Penguin, 2008.

8. Weir, K., "Forgiveness Can Improve Mental and Physical Health," *American Psychological Association*, *48*(1), 2017.

9. Warrier, V., et al., "Elevated Rates of Autism, Other Neurodevelopmental and Psychiatric Diagnoses, and Autistic Traits in Transgender and Gender-Diverse Individuals," *Nature Communications*, 11(1), 2020, 3959.

10. Some neurotypicals can misunderstand an autistic person's fascination with odd and possibly morbid subject matter, like true crime or school shootings, which Madrid referred to. This is usually not a reflection of their intentions or a dark personality. It is usually just an interest that happens to be odd or creepy to some people, possibly stemming from a broader interest in psychology and understanding other people intellectually, though this is deeply speculative.

11. Marshall, E., et al., "Non-suicidal Self-Injury and Suicidality in Trans People: A Systematic Review of the Literature," *International Review of Psychiatry*, 28(1), 2016, 58–69.

12. Birmingham, E., et al., "Implicit Social Biases in People with Autism," *Psychological Science*, 26(11), 2015, 1693–1705.

13. Ratto, A.B., et al., "What About the Girls? Sex-Based Differences in Autistic Traits and Adaptive Skills," *Journal of Autism and Developmental Disorders*, 48(5), 2018, 1698–711.

14. Kanner, L., and L. Lesser, "Early Infantile Autism," *Pediatric Clinics of North America*, 5, 1958, 711–30.

15. Loomes, R., L. Hull, and WP.L. Mandy, "What Is the Male-to-Female Ratio in Autism Spectrum Disorder? A Systematic Review and Meta-Analysis," *Journal of the American Academy of Child and Adolescent Psychiatry*, 56(6), 2017, 466–74.

16. Werling, D.M., and D.H. Geschwind, "Sex Differences in Autism Spectrum Disorders, *Current Opinion in Neurology*, 26(2), 2013, 146–53.

17. Giarelli, E., et al., "Sex Differences in the Evaluation and Diagnosis of Autism Spectrum Disorders Among Children," *Disability and Health Journal*, 3(2), 2010, 107–16; Bargiela, S., R. Steward, and W. Mandy, "The Experiences of Late-diagnosed Women with Autism Spectrum Conditions: An Investigation of the Female Autism Phenotype," *Journal of Autism and Developmental Disorders*, 46(10), 2016, 3281–94.

18. Cazalis, F., et al., "Evidence that Nine Autistic Women out of Ten Have Been Victims of Sexual Violence," *Frontiers in Behavioral Neuroscience*, 16, 2022, 852203.

19. Name has been changed for privacy reasons.

20. Baron-Cohen, S., *The Essential Difference: Male and Female Brains and the Truth About Autism,* Basic Books, 2004, 8.

21. Baron-Cohen, S. "The Extreme Male Brain Theory of Autism," *Trends in Cognitive Sciences*, 6(6), 2002, 248–54.

22. Chopra, S., et al., "Gender Differences in Undergraduate Engineering Applicants: A Text Mining Approach," Paper presented at International Educational Data Mining (EDM) Conference, July 16, 2018. Retrieved November 21, 2022, from https://files.eric.ed.gov; Vere-Jones, E. "Why Are There So Few Men in Nursing?" *Nursing Times*, March 3, 2008. Retrieved November 22, 2022, from www.nursingtimes.net; Ubando, M., "Gender Differences in Intimacy, Emotional Expressivity, and Relationship Satisfaction," *Pepperdine Journal of Communication Research*, 4(1), 2016, 13.

23. Baron-Cohen, *The Essential Difference,* 154.

24. Generation Next, *Could It Be Asperger's?*, video, January 25, 2015, www.youtube.com/watch?v=LuZFThlOiJI

25. Becerra, T.A., et al., "Autism Spectrum Disorders and Race, Ethnicity, and Nativity: A Population-Based Study," *Pediatrics*, 134(1), 2014, e63–e71. 8

26. Gemegah, Hartas, and Totsika, "Public Attitudes to People with ASD."

27. Autism Women's Network, *All the Weight of Our Dreams: On Living Racialized Autism*, DragonBee Press, 2017, 496, 498.

28. Ibid.

29. Zeliadt, N., "School Survey in India Reveals Low Autism Prevalence," *Spectrum*, July 12, 2017. Retrieved November 12, 2022, from www.spectrumnews.org

30. Giwa Onaiwu, M., "'They Don't Know, Don't Show, or Don't Care': Autism's White Privilege Problem," *Autism in Adulthood*, *2*(4), 2017.

31. Kanner, "Autistic Disturbances," 218–219.

32. Clay, R.A., "Women Outnumber Men in Psychology, but Not in the Field's Top Echelons," *American Psychological Association*, *48*(7), 2017, 18.

33. Center for Disease Control, *Spotlight On: Racial and Ethnic Differences in Children Identified with Autism Spectrum Disorder (ASD)*, n.d. Retrieved November 21, 2022, from https://www.cdc.gov/ncbddd/autism/addm-community-report/differences-in-children.html

34. Hendrickx, S., *Love, Sex, & Long-Term Relationships*, Jessica Kingsley, 2008, 85.

35. Velten, J., and J. Margraf, "Satisfaction Guaranteed? How Individual, Partner, and Relationship Factors Impact Sexual Satisfaction within Partnerships," *PLOS ONE*, 12(2), 2017, e0172855.

36. Hendrickx, *Love, Sex, & Long-Term Relationships*, 84.

37. Carley, *Asperger's from the Inside Out*, 193.

38. Ibid., "Introduction."

39. "Supporting Happy and Positive Sexual Lives," *Uniquely Human: The Podcast*, April 16, 2021. Retrieved November 19, 2022, from https://uniquelyhuman.com/2021/04/16/supporting-happy-and-positive-sexual-lives-michael-john-carley/

40. Ibid.

41. Weiss, J.A., and M.A. Fardella, "Victimization and Perpetration Experiences of Adults with Autism," *Frontiers in Psychiatry*, 9, 2018, 203.

42. Attwood, T., *The Complete Guide to Asperger's Syndrome*, 2nd ed., Jessica Kingsley Publishers, 2015, 100.

43. Solomon, D., D.W. Pantalone, and S. Faja, "Autism and Adult Sex Education: A Literature Review Using the Information-Motivation-Behavioral Skills Framework," *Sexuality and Disability*, 37(3), 2019, 339–51.

44. Lowinger, S., and S. Pearlman-Avnion, *Autism in Adulthood*, Springer, 2019, 209.

45. Weir, E., C. Allison, and S. Baron-Cohen, "The Sexual Health, Orientation, and Activity of Autistic Adolescents and Adults," *Autism Research*, *14*(11), 2021, 2342–54.

46. Lowinger and Pearlman-Avnion, *Autism in Adulthood*, 46.

47. Howlin, *Autism and Asperger Syndrome*, 325; Lowinger and Pearlman-Avnion, *Autism in Adulthood*, 209.

48. Kurchak, S., 'I'm Autistic. I Just Turned 36, the Average Age When People Like Me Die," *Vox*, February 19, 2018; Bennie, M., 'The Three Main Causes of Early Death in Autism," Autism Awareness Centre Inc. (blog), April 18, 2016. Retrieved November 21, 2022, from https://autismawarenesscentre.com

49. Bilder, D., et al., "Excess Mortality and Causes of Death in Autism Spectrum Disorders: A Follow Up of the 1980s Utah/UCLA Autism Epidemiologic Study," *Journal of Autism and Developmental Disorders*, 43(5), 2013, 1196–204; Hirvikoski, T., et al., "Premature Mortality in Autism Spectrum Disorder," *British Journal of Psychiatry*, 208(3), 2016, 232–38.

50. Wright, J., 'The Link Between Epilepsy and Autism, Explained," *Spectrum*, October 21, 2019. Retrieved November 21, 2022, from www.spectrumnews.org; Center for Disease Control, *Epilepsy Data and Statistics*, n.d. Retrieved November 21, 2022, from https://www.cdc.gov/epilepsy/data/

51. Marcus Autism Center, *What To Do When Your Child Elopes*, n.d. Retrieved November 22, 2022, from https://www.marcus.org/autism-resources/autism-tips-and-resources/what-to-do-when-your-child-elopes

52. Smith DaWalt, L., et al., "Mortality in Individuals with Autism Spectrum Disorder: Predictors Over a 20-Year Period," *Autism: The International Journal of Research and Practice*, 23(7), 2019, 1732–39.

53. Volkmar, Reichow, and McPartland, *Adolescents and Adults with Autism Spectrum Disorders*, 217.

54. South, M., A.P. Costa, and C. McMorris, "Death by Suicide Among People with Autism: Beyond Zebrafish," *JAMA Network Open*, 4(1), 2021, e2034018.

55. Autistica, *Suicide and Autism*, n.d. Retrieved November 22, 2022, from https://www.autistica.org.uk/what-is-autism/signs-and-symptoms/suicide-and-autism

56. Celano, C.M., et al., "Anxiety Disorders and Cardiovascular Disease," *Current Psychiatry Reports*, 18(11), 2016, 101; Horn, P.J., and L.A. Wuyek, "Anxiety Disorders as a Risk Factor for Subsequent Depression," *International Journal of Psychiatry in Clinical Practice*, 14(4), 2010, 244–47.

57. Koegel, R.L., and M. Mentis, "Motivation in Childhood Autism: Can They or Won't They?" *Journal of Child Psychology and Psychiatry, and Allied Disciplines*, 26(2), 1985, 185–91.

58. Mohammadi, M.R., et al., "Prevalence of Autism and Its Comorbidities and the Relationship with Maternal Psychopathology: A National Population-Based Study," *Archives of Iranian Medicine*, 22, 2019, 546–53.

59. Not his real name.

60. National Institute of Mental Health, *Any Anxiety Disorder*, n.d. Retrieved November 19, 2022, from https://www.nimh.nih.gov/health/statistics/any-anxiety-disorder

61. Vasa, R.A., and M.O. Mazurek, "An Update on Anxiety in Youth with Autism Spectrum Disorders," *Current Opinion in Psychiatry*, 28(2), 2015, 83–90.

62. Bloch, C., et al., "Alexithymia Traits Outweigh Autism Traits in the Explanation of Depression in Adults with Autism," *Nature: Scientific Reports, 11,* 2021, 2258.

63. Generation Next, *Could It Be Asperger's?*

64. Gravitz, L., "Does Autism Raise the Risk of PTSD?" *Scientific American*, October 1, 2018.

65. Stoddart, K., L. Burke, and R. King., *Asperger Syndrome in Adulthood: A Comprehensive Guide for Clinicians*, W.W. Norton, 2012, 101; National Autistic Society, *Distinguishing Between Autism & Abuse*, Video, May 8, 2015, www.youtube.com/watch?v=I0TUIMWWVIE

66. LeClerc, S., and D. Easley, "Pharmacological Therapies for Autism Spectrum Disorder: A Review," *Pharmacy and Therapeutics,* 40(6), 2015, 389–97.

67. Geggel, L. "Ritalin Probe," *Spectrum*, July 16, 2013. Retrieved November 21, 2022, from www.spectrumnews.org; PsychCentral, *Medications for Autism Spectrum Disorder*, n.d. Retrieved November 21, 2022, from https://psychcentral.com

68. Stoddart, Burke, and King, *Asperger Syndrome in Adulthood*, 220–21.
69. Ibid.
70. Weir, E., C. Allison, and S. Baron-Cohen, "Understanding the Substance Use of Autistic Adolescents and Adults: A Mixed-Methods Approach," *The Lancet*.
71. Ibid.
72. Lowinger and Pearlman-Avnion, *Autism in Adulthood*, 42.
73. Ibid.
74. Heeramun, R,. et al., "Autism and Convictions for Violent Crimes: Population-Based Cohort Study in Sweden," *Journal of the American Academy of Child & Adolescent Psychiatry*, 56(6), 2017, 491.
75. National Autistic Society, *Criminal Justice: A Guide for Police Officers and Professionals*. Retrieved November 21, 2022, from https://www.autism.org.uk/advice-and-guidance/topics/criminal-justice/criminal-justice/professionals
76. Calton, S., and G. Hall, "Autistic Adults and Their Experiences with Police Personnel: A Qualitative Inquiry," *Psychiatry, Psychology, and Law*, 29(2), 2021, 274–89.
77. Ibid
78. Chiacchia, M., "Autism Spectrum Disorder and the Criminal Justice System," *Purdue Global* (blog), April 5, 2016. Retrieved November 21, 2022, from https://www.purdueglobal.edu
79. ABC News In Depth, *Is Asperger's Syndrome the Next Stage of Human Evolution?: Tony Attwood*, Video, September 25, 2017, www.youtube.com/watch?v=vdQDvLXLqiM
80. Attwood, W., *Asperger's Syndrome and Jail*, Jessica Kingsley, 2018.
81. Ibid.
82. Ibid.
83. Collins, J., et al., "A Systematic Review of Autistic People and the Criminal Justice System: An Update of King and Murphy (2014)," *Journal of Autism and Developmental Disorders*, 53(8), 2023, 3151-79.
84. ABC News In Depth, *Is Asperger's Syndrome the Next Stage of Human Evolution?*

## Conclusion

1. ABC News, *GMA: Autistic Pride, June 10, 2008*, https://www.youtube.com/watch?v=oouMQG3Oh6c
2. AutismCareUK, *Prof. Tony Attwood in Conversation with Autism Care UK*, Video, May 25, 2012, https://youtu.be/nJTl1dyL1zs

# INDEX

## ABOUT THE AUTHOR

After graduating from the University of Toronto in 2014, Daniel Smeenk started his career in journalism working as a copy editor and book reviewer for Brunswick News Inc. in Saint John, New Brunswick, before becoming a reporter for Great West Newspapers in northern Alberta. Since 2018, Daniel Smeenk has worked in public relations. He is autistic, passionate about sports, music, and social science–type subjects, and lives in St. Catharines, Ontario.